GLOBAL HEALTH
MEANS LISTENING

ALSO BY RAYMOND DOWNING

The Wedding Goes On Without Us, including Bury Me Naked

As They See It: The Development of the African AIDS Discourse

*Suffering and Healing in America: An American Doctor's
View from the Outside*

Death and Life in America: Biblical Healing and Biomedicine

Biohealth: Beyond Medicalization, Imposing Health

Such a Time of It They Had: Global Health Pioneers in Africa

Global Health
Means Listening

Raymond Downing, MD

MANQA
books

NAIROBI

Published by Manqa Books
www.manqa.net

Editing by Edward Miller
Cover and book design by Edward Miller

First Edition
10 9 8 7 6 5

To Harold Miller, who first told me to listen and showed me how

and

To Prof. Barasa Otsyula, to whom I still listen

Understanding global poverty...requires listening to those affected by poverty, which is to say the poor and otherwise marginalized. Listening is also a significant part of accompaniment, and of clinical medicine. Listening is thus both engagement and research.

The self-styled liberators from poverty are too often those who want to preach, rather than listen, to the poor. The theme of receptive hearing as linked to humility runs throughout Father Gutierrez's work as both pastor and theologian: "Working in this world [of the poor] and becoming familiar with it, I came to realize, together with others, the first thing to do is to listen."

Listening carefully is hard to do.

When we actually went out and did what we said we were doing, which was listening to the poor, we discovered that we weren't listening enough.*

—Paul Farmer

*From M. Griffin and J. W. Block, editors, *In the Company of the Poor: Conversations between Dr. Paul Farmer and Father Gustavo Gutierrez* (Maryknoll, New York: Orbis Books, 2013).

Introduction

AT THE BEGINNING of this century, international health development refashioned itself with a new name: Global Health. "Why is that term so attractive to so many?" a colleague working with Partners In Health wondered. "It is almost as though the very words unlocked this reservoir of energy and passion that was not there before—especially thinking of the many young idealistic people now working in PIH."[1] It's more than a name change. The rapid growth in interest among students, in graduate programs being developed, and in funding available for new initiatives all indicate a convergence toward a universally accepted goal: good health for the entire world's population.

This is surely a hopeful movement in a world torn by inequity. The "end poverty" and "zero hunger" slogans may be over the top, but working toward these goals has got to be useful—especially when Christians and Muslims, conservatives and liberals, Africans and Asians and Westerners are all pulling in the same direction. As with world peace, or saving the earth, we seem to have found another global good.

So I decided to contribute my experience. I have been working in global health in Africa for 30 years. I was interim manager of a refugee health program in eastern Sudan in the 1980s. I worked in a mission hospital in

Tanzania in the 1990s where I did community health surveys and helped start a mosquito net distribution program—and did the medical and surgical work in the hospital. In 1994 I was director of the new medical department for a council of churches in southern Sudan during the war there. I returned to mission hospital work in Kenya for the rest of the 1990s. Then for the last decade I have been on the faculty of Moi University School of Medicine, helping to develop the first family medicine training program in Kenya.

In all of this, I have learned many theories and written many words. In trying to make some sense out of all this experience, I collected some three dozen of the essays I had written during this time and read them over together. I found a theme running through many of them: the need to listen—listen to the past, listen to colleagues, listen to our faith, but mostly listen to the people we have come to serve. Listen. Learn.

"Listening and learning" was a mantra I picked up 30 years ago when we started working with the Mennonite Central Committee. As I listened to what Africans told me about their customs and how those traditions influenced health and healing, I began to wonder if health development could be rooted in African experience, and how we could build on the wisdom there. Listening and learning seemed like such good advice then, and still does now.

But global health is not set up to find the way people

used to do things and ask what was good about that; neither were its precursors. Missionary medicine's clear goal was to save souls. Tropical medicine set out to find the biomedical causes of diseases its practitioners confronted. International health development tried to control or eradicate those diseases. The unstated assumption for global health, as for its precursors, is "we have what they need."

Nevertheless, global health does listen—but now to statistics more than to people. Statistics, we say, are a way to find out what the real problems are, objectively. We count parasites and measure heights and weights and record hospital admissions and births and deaths. And then, using statistically analyzed opinion surveys, we can find out what everyone thinks. If there is a great variety, we can at least discover what the average person thinks (if we are steeped in statistical thinking) or what the majority thinks (if we are steeped in democratic thinking).

Then, based on what the statistics say, and rooted in an unquestioned loyalty to the methods and products of biomedicine, global health chooses a goal. Yes, we—we professionals—choose the goal. We then find an evidence-based "best practice" to get there, set up an efficient model, obtain community buy-in, build capacity, and plan for sustainability. As the pilot studies show statistics improving, we scale up, publish our findings, and hope others will learn from this evidence.

If this is global health, I began to doubt whether listening to people made any sense any more. Perhaps we were beyond the time when listening to traditional ways of doing things would be helpful, when there was any chance for development to be rooted in African realities. If health only means lowering mortality rates—if global health is only a grand exercise in improving statistics—then we don't need to listen. Give the technicians and entrepreneurs free reign.

This makes sense if the objects of global health are only mosquitoes and bacteria, or wells and latrines, or schools and diplomas, or yields per acre and dollars per day. But ultimately the objects of global health are subjects: people. If only because humans deserve the dignity of having a voice, we must listen to them.

But it is far more than dignity. Global health has the opportunity to expand its knowledge base significantly by listening to ancient and indigenous wisdom. It can enhance known interventions by listening to the priorities of local people. Global health can help to ensure its relevance and effectiveness by continuing to monitor not just what happens to people, but especially what those people think about what's happening to them. In other words, listen.

Is it possible for global health, as an enterprise, to listen to what people think and want, and blend its expertise with that? Or is it too late?

In writing this book, I have chosen to believe it is not too late. Using those three dozen random and sporadic essays—that is, using my experience—as a starting point, I decided to present a single extended argument about why we in global health must listen.

Part I contains some stories and reflections on global health. None of these chapters is a pure academic exercise: each one contains my reflections about an experience I had, a conference I went to, a question I was asked, a book I read. I am not attempting a new definition of global health, but more a series of commentaries on definitions I have absorbed.

The next two parts contain my reflections on global health areas in which I have worked. Part II is about AIDS. My work here was not in an antiretroviral clinic treating AIDS patients—though as a doctor working in East African hospitals I have examined and treated many patients with AIDS. Rather, my focus here is on how Africans see this epidemic. As many of these reflections are drawn from research I did in preparation for a book (*As They See It: The Development of the African AIDS Discourse*), they are in a more academic style.

Part III contains parallel reflections on the development of family medicine. I have spent the last decade working in an academic family medicine department in an African university, helping to initiate the first family medicine training program in Kenya. While the setting is formally academic, much of what goes on in academic departments is bureaucracy, dealing with donors, and strife. I had expected a scholarly environment and did the necessary background reading—and research—for an academic task. I spent most of my time trying to keep my head above water. What I have included here is further reflections on listening and learning in this environment.

Part IV goes in a different direction. Part of my career has been as a "medical missionary," supported by American Mennonite or Quaker congregations. Medical missionaries were some of the first global health workers and continue to contribute significantly to global health—though many of us prefer terms such as "Christian development worker" connoting service, rather than "medical missionary" connoting evangelism. The spiritual foundation that we share is my interest, and my reflections here focus on what our biblical faith says about listening and healing and suffering and our presence in this God-soaked continent.

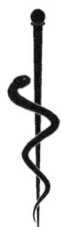

PART I:
GLOBAL HEALTH

1. Bury Me Naked

I WILL BEGIN with some stories about some friends of mine, an anesthetist named Onyango and a surgeon named Wafula, from a hospital I worked at in western Kenya—only those aren't their real names. I want to tell you some very personal things about them, things which might embarrass them or their families. But it is sometimes the very personal things which reveal our deepest truths and our most profound wisdom. I want to begin this book with some of the wisdom which they, by accepting my friendship, revealed to me. The core of global health is listening to and learning from stories like these.

Several years ago students were rioting in Nairobi—it might have been because they didn't like the food in the dining halls. One day I was discussing these riots with Dr. Wafula, a local surgeon, and he gave me this enigmatic explanation for the riots: "I can't talk to my father." I knew he wasn't lamenting his own version of the generation gap, but I didn't understand what that had to do with student riots. I needed his point spelled out, so he spelled it out for me.

The students, he said, did not know how to communicate directly and yet politely with their elders, because in African culture children do not talk directly to their fathers about important matters. So when frustration grows and there is no way to let it out, students riot. It goes the other way too, he said. Fathers don't talk directly to their children: the administration did not negotiate with the students, it closed the university.

By now Onyango, the anesthetist, was in on the conversation, and we were getting away from the students. "But we do talk to our mothers," they both agreed. The mother, they said, is the mediator. I go to my mother with a difficult matter, and she talks to my father, then brings the answer back. Not immediately, and not by appointment. The time has to be right, but my father will eventually respond to my needs: he must, he's my father.

It wasn't long after this that we had a chance to see what this all meant, not for students in the university, but for Dr. Wafula and Dr. Muroto, an older colleague of his. Both are Kenyan-trained general surgeons: Muroto more serious and better trained in the early postcolonial days; Wafula younger, more jovial, eager to learn. We had consulted Dr. Wafula on a very difficult orthopedic case with several arm and leg fractures needing operative repair. He felt it was beyond his ability and suggested we refer the patient elsewhere. But when the family asked Dr. Muroto's opinion, he said he could do it—except that Dr. Wafula had already been consulted, so he could not interfere.

No problem, we thought. We'll just see if Dr. Wafula would agree to do the case with Muroto, the older surgeon.

He agreed—but there was a problem. The arrangements just weren't getting made, and the patient lay in ineffective traction for three, four, five, six weeks. Whenever we'd see Wafula, he'd say that he just missed seeing Muroto, or he was out, or this week wasn't good because of other cases one or the other of them had. But Wafula had already explained to us this difficulty of communicating with his elder: "I can't talk to my father."

It was a problem, but this time knowing what the problem was told us how to solve it. Onyango saw the patient lying in bed every day, running up his bill, not getting better, and he decided to do something. He knew both surgeons well and had their respect: both surgeons agreed to operate at our hospital because we had supplies, a good nursing staff—and Onyango. He was in a position to be the mediator, to be the mother. So he set to work.

One Saturday a week or two later, Onyango gave the anesthesia, and the two surgeons operated for eight hours. A couple of weeks later, the patient walked home.

A few years later, the students were rioting in Nairobi again. Shortly before the riots started, a young man came in with his femur fractured in several places. We put him in temporary traction, but said the best treatment would be surgery to insert a plate and screws to hold the bone in place. He brought in a deposit; we bought the plate and screws; we called Dr. Wafula. We were all ready for surgery—and then Dr. Wafula said that this was a particularly difficult fracture, and he'd like the older surgeon to help him.

Funny thing: he had trouble contacting him. He either just missed him at the office, or his phone wasn't working, or he wasn't home. Two weeks after the patient had brought in the deposit, we still hadn't operated. Or perhaps: only two weeks had passed when Wafula finally got through to Muroto. We agreed to begin at eight o'clock on a Saturday morning. When I arrived at the hospital at a couple minutes past eight, Wafula was just arriving—and Muroto had already come, had felt things weren't ready, and had left in a huff.

I was angry and embarrassed, because the patient was on my ward, and I had to face him. But my anger is irrelevant to this story. Wafula said he would consult with Muroto. Sunday night he called and said they would do the case Tuesday afternoon at two. On Tuesday I was in the parking lot by a quarter till two. Onyango was waiting—Muroto came, then Wafula came, and together they walked into the operating theater.

Four hours later the case was finished, the older surgeon had left, and Wafula was finishing up, grinning. "How did it go?" I asked.

"Wonderful," he said. "One more like that and I'll be able to do it alone."

"But how did things go with the *mzee*—the older

surgeon?" I asked. "Wasn't this another example of how you couldn't talk to your father?"

"No," he said, "when my father is angry, I leave him alone for a while, then I go back when he has calmed down and I ask him gently what I need."

"Fine," I answered, not satisfied, still feeling my own anger, still trying to understand. "But how could you be so sure that the *mzee* would eventually help you? Why should your elder listen to you then?"

"He can't refuse me," said Wafula. "He's my father."

*

Are we in the global health industry listening to stories like these? Do we understand the hierarchies in the cultures where we work, the communication patterns, the ways that people themselves get things done? There is a pace in Africa which is different: slower, almost antithetical to the pace we learn in emergency departments. Can we slow down? Do we appreciate indigenous mediation techniques, or are we still trying to teach health management—as we understand it—to local people?

Did you hear the story of the Kenyan diplomat who saved the South Africa elections in 1994? One faction, a Zulu ethnic group, was refusing to participate in the election, threatening the entire anti-apartheid process. An international diplomatic delegation, including prominent names from the USA and UK—I think Kissinger was one of them—tried to convince the leader, Chief Buthelezi, to participate, but failed completely. The chief left, the English and American diplomats left, but there was a Kenyan diplomat who stayed on. Then Buthelezi's plane had some engine trouble and he had to turn around—and found the Kenyan waiting. Now they could talk, African to African, about their own issues, at their own pace. Buthelezi agreed to participate in the election, and the rest is history. Can we get a glimpse that African culture might have something to teach us?

These questions are seminal, but they are not the sort of questions an industry usually asks of itself. Our job is to produce something, and at a stretch we'll ask questions like these if they help us to produce a better product, more efficiently. Have we who work in the healing arts— whether in Africa or the USA—become so infected by the market that we really believe health is something that can be packaged and distributed?

*

As I was preparing these stories for publication, together with others like them that illustrate the remarkable resilience of Africans in the face of suffering, I discovered an old, mostly abandoned burial custom of the Luhya people of western Kenya where I was working. John Mbiti, a revered Kenyan philosopher and theologian, says this: "The body is buried facing west, and completely naked just as the person was when he was born. This 'naked' state symbolizes birth into the hereafter. Stripping the corpse and burying it completely naked is a concrete externalization of the concept of death as birth into the hereafter." At birth, Mbiti is saying, people leave the spirit world and come to live among humans; at death, they return to the spirit world. In Africa, death is not the opposite of life, it is merely the end of life…or so I wrote in an essay about suffering and healing in Africa. But a friend, a Kenyan university lecturer, corrected me after reading that essay. Death is not even the end of life, he said. Life goes on with the living dead, with the ancestors.

It all makes so much sense to me, this African understanding of living and dying. It makes sense because it fits with and feeds my Christian beliefs. It makes sense because it illuminates Onyango and Wafula's profound insights; they have a longer view than we in the West. It makes sense because it leads to hope.

I had stumbled on an obscure custom, one that had apparently died out but that had such rich meaning: death is simply birth into the hereafter. *Human life on earth is not all of life*. One reason for African hope in the middle of bleeding and suffering and dying is that Africa knows that bleeding and suffering and dying are not sovereign.

So I decided: even though no one else does it, when I die, bury me naked.

*

When I first showed a draft of my book *Bury Me Naked* to Onyango, his immediate response surprised me: "So you want to be buried naked. Did you put that in your will?" Since Onyango and other friends found the idea of being buried naked humorous, his question to me was posed in a joking manner, and I felt no obligation to answer seriously.

But his question bothered me. At first I thought he missed my point: being buried naked is a metaphor, and he was taking my title far too literally. Before I had become comfortable with this response, however, I realized the depth of his question. I was trying to celebrate an African understanding of living and dying, a view of the world very different from my own, and Onyango was simply asking how serious I was. Did I really think African customs, and the meaning behind them, were superior to my own? Was I serious about integrating them into my life? Would this even be possible?

Onyango often made me think, asking questions that stuck with me. Not long after this discussion, we had another—a bit more difficult for me because it was during a C-section. It began, I think, as I was about to cut the skin. Onyango was wondering how I would translate the Swahili word *heshima*. I sliced, and the flesh fell apart, first glistening yellow fat, then blood from cut veins running between the globules. "Respect," I said without much thought, and I kept cutting. Onyango wasn't satisfied; he felt that "honor" was a better word. I was by now cutting into the uterus and blood welled up into the incision site. I couldn't see if I'd gotten through yet and stabbed again, worried that I'd slice the baby. The baby was big, face up (ah, so that's why it wouldn't deliver!), and fortunately had no lacerations. I removed it without difficulty, but had lost the thread of the discussion.

Onyango hadn't. What's the difference between honor and respect? he asked. I hadn't thought about it before, and now thinking, sewing the first layer of the uterus, I realized that I wanted respect, but didn't care about honor. That in fact I had some idea about what respect was, but wasn't sure at all I knew what honor was. I was nearing the end of the second layer when Onyango said that he would prefer to be honored. I had trouble right then wondering why, because bright red blood started pumping where I was sewing.

Just put in a few deep sutures, he said in between respect and honor. I did, but it kept oozing. He said "Put in a figure-of-eight stitch there" at the same time as I said "Call Dr. Juma," my boss—and I won, because I was the one with the needle and thread, and I stopped sewing and put pressure on the bleeding place and waited. After Dr. Juma came and left (his contribution being to put in a figure-of-eight stitch, which stopped the bleeding), Onyango told me why he preferred to be honored. Because God honors us, he said; it says so in Isaiah. Chapter 43.

Two days later I asked Dr. Wafula how he would translate *heshima*. Honor, he said. And which would he prefer—to be honored or respected? Honored, he said—but you in America, he said, you have a better idea about honor than us. Where, I wondered, does that fit with my sense that America has at least some memory of what respect means but views honor mostly as a quaint medieval remnant? Well, he said, look at the way you treat your famous people.

Oh. My confusion began to clear. Yes, I told him, how we treat famous people has all of the form of honor, but none of the substance. We inflate whatever real qualities they might have, like blowing up a balloon with a picture on it, and the more we fill the balloon with emptiness, the more the picture distorts. Then we look for the opportunity to pop it.

Ah, he said, I see. You elevate someone, but rejoice when they fall—but when God honors us, He wants to lift us up when we fall.

*

On Good Friday 2001, Friday the thirteenth, my wife Jan, our son Tim, and I were watching a video at our house—*Children of a Lesser God*. Dr. Juma's wife Consolata came to the door. I paused the video and went to the bathroom while Jan talked with Consolata. As I was coming out, Jan met me in the hall. "Ray, Onyango's dead."

"WHAT?"

"Just what I said, Onyango's dead."

"You're joking."

"Why would I joke about something like that?"

"Oh…no…Oh my goodness. Oh, oh…."

For several years, Onyango was our only anesthetist—meaning he was on call all the time, day and night. We did occasionally arrange for locums to substitute for him, and by mid-2000 we had finally hired a second anesthetist, Ezekiel. His presence gave Onyango a chance to take a long-postponed annual leave in January 2001. Many skilled hospital employees use their annual leaves to work elsewhere and make extra money. Normally Onyango would have done the same. But this year I doubt it entered his mind; this year he was going to work on his farm. A few years before he had bought two acres of land in the "schemes"—excellent farmland developed into large plantations by white farmers in the colonial days, and then divided at independence into smaller plots and offered for sale.

Onyango was very bright. He did well in primary

school—until the person paying his school fees died and he had to drop out. He eventually entered nursing school, but again did not finish. The provincial surgeon—the same older surgeon Wafula operated with—found out about him and helped him to get a year-long training course in anesthesia, then suggested he go to our mission hospital to work.

But in the last year or two, it was farming that was in the front of his mind. He planted maize every year and kept a couple of cows. A brother stayed at the farm to look after it, but whenever he had the chance he'd go—to treat a sick cow or help with the weeding or harvest the maize. He wasn't the only farmer working at the hospital. Most staff members supplemented their meager hospital salaries by growing food—even the doctors.

We didn't see Onyango much in January: he had taken his annual leave. I had heard rumors that he had a new wife and a new baby, but he hadn't mentioned anything to me. I did know, though, that he had had quite a bit of difficulty with his previous wife. They were together when we first met in 1995, with a small child just old enough to be scared of me. That wife washed floors in the hospital and was very quiet. I didn't know much about their relationship until it became unpleasant. He never told me why, but eventually her family stepped in and removed the children (they had had a second one by then). Onyango and his wife separated, but both continued working at the hospital.

When Onyango returned from his leave, I asked how his harvest was. Good, he said. Very good. In fact—he took me aside to tell me this—he had used the profits to buy a tractor. It was a secondhand tractor and cost, I eventually found out, 550,000 Kenya shillings—almost 8,000 dollars—and Onyango had paid the owner 400,000 of that. He was excited, and nervous, about his new purchase.

The first time I saw his tractor was a few weeks later when it was near the hospital to be repaired: a big blue Ford tractor with huge front wheels. "Is it four-wheel drive?" I asked. "Yes—but something doesn't work, so we disconnected the driveshaft from the front wheels." It was then that he told me that there was another critical part that had broken, and he needed 10,000 shillings to fix it. But as soon as it was fixed, he assured me, he could plow with it and repay me.

By now Onyango was back at the hospital, and sharing the work with Ezekiel allowed him more time to farm—or, now, to try to get his tractor fixed. He was so good with his work that it was no stress for him; he even came to work once with malaria, gave the appropriate anesthesia, and sat draped over his anesthesia machine—still monitoring the patient adequately. After his malaria was treated, he was back to his usual joking self, dancing with me in the operating room, calling me Chuck Norris (I called him Eddie Murphy), making me laugh even when we were both called for an operation in the middle of the night.

His farm, though, continued to be a source of problems. Someone stole his cow, then the tractor driver got drunk and drove it without enough oil in the engine. He borrowed money from several friends, and continued to build up debts with the tractor repair company that eventually reached over 90,000 shillings. The money problems involved his family as well. His new wife's sister had borrowed some money and wasn't returning it. And his mother had severe high blood pressure, with her medicines costing most of his monthly paycheck from the hospital. Just her medicines.

Around this time we had a brief conversation in front of the hospital, another one of those that stuck with me. We were talking about my upcoming return to the USA for an extended time, this time to work and make some money, and Onyango began reflecting on how much he could make if he lived in the States. Though I have heard this assertion often—and equally often want to respond, "It's not that easy"—with Onyango I believed it. If he had had the opportunity for a US education, or even just a green card, he would have much more money. But he didn't ask me for help in getting a US green card. After toying only briefly with self-pity, he quoted to me a Swahili proverb, one I hadn't heard before: "The One who gives you a chair is the same One who gives me a grass mat." The grass mat, he explained, was where the older people in the house sat—mats like these being readily available and cheap. The chair was something more modern, something costly. The mat was a symbol of tradition; the chair of wealth. Both were gifts from the same God.

Holy Week came. Onyango was getting more upset with his wife, and with her sister not returning the money. He told a friend he was considering leaving his wife. His tractor broke again.

On Tuesday, Dr. Juma's main operating day, I found Onyango in the operating room as usual, helping Ezekiel. I came looking for him because I had just been called to see two children who were unconscious, but I wasn't sure why. I told him the symptoms, and he came directly to the pediatric ward. The father had given both children what he thought was worm medicine—because it was in a worm medicine bottle—but they both got violently ill. Onyango smelled the medicine from the bottle and knew immediately it was concentrated cattle dip insecticide—a terrible mistake. Several of us were working to resuscitate the children, but we were too late for the younger one, an eight-year-old girl. We gave the other, an eleven-year-old boy, the appropriate antidote, and he began waking up. Onyango looked energized, the way he always did in critical situations, helping to bring someone back from the brink. I discharged the boy two days later.

On Wednesday Onyango said he needed to sort out the problem with the stolen cow. It had been found butchered, and he was going to the village authorities

to do what was necessary to get it replaced. He also succeeded in finally getting his tractor fixed, and on Thursday
it plowed in a nearby village. On Friday it broke again. He
saw the tractor, told his brother to bring it to the service
station, and then went from the hospital up to his farm in
the schemes. His wife also went, and they argued there.
He told her he wanted the money from her sister; she said
she was leaving him. She then took their infant and left.
About midday he called Dr. Wafula, but Wafula wasn't in.

On Friday evening at about sundown, Onyango's
brother came to the hospital and asked for the ambulance.
Four people from the hospital went. A couple hours later
Consolata, Dr. Juma's wife, was knocking at our door
while we were watching *Children of a Lesser God*.

*

Why would a young man of 36 suddenly die? Did he get
some unknown rapidly progressing disease? Was he hit
by a car? Did one of his creditors, or one of his wives,
murder him? Or did he kill himself? Those questions were
disturbingly easy to answer. On Thursday Ezekiel found
five ampules of pancuronium missing from the anesthetic
drug cabinet. Pancuronium does not anesthetize—it
simply rapidly paralyzes all muscles, including those
needed for breathing. On Friday evening those who went
in the ambulance to pick up Onyango found no signs

of a struggle, no marks on his body, and a broken pan-curonium ampule, a needle, and a syringe in the room. No one in the hospital had suspected that Onyango was near the edge—but neither did anyone doubt that he had taken his own life.

But why did he do it? Albert, one of those who went to get his body, told me the next day, "It was the tractor." Wafula said, "I knew he had financial problems. Everyone does. Things are bad in Kenya." But two other people told us, "People don't kill themselves just because of money problems." Dr. Juma was convinced it was the difficulties with his wife. "He had a serious dispute with his wife that very morning that he killed himself," he told me. "When you don't have a stable family, things are bad." And the provincial surgeon told us that even he felt responsible, because he had been the one to provide him with the training that ultimately gave him the tools to take his own life. Maybe it was all these things. The economy in Africa *is* bad; people *do* have relationship problems. But Onyango wasn't starving, he was climbing—or trying to climb. Instead he was spinning those big tractor wheels in the mud, spraying it all over the place, getting nowhere.

How could the one who mediated between two surgeons fail to seek a mediator? How could the man who reminded me that his grass mat was from the same One who gave me the chair—how could he get so involved with the chair? Onyango was buried in a locally made wooden casket with a glass window and a hinged lid over the upper third of his body. His body was wrapped in a white cloth. After the ceremony and hymns, six hospital workers carried his casket through the crowd to the gravesite and lowered it in. Then "Ashes to ashes, dust to dust…," and the first handful of dirt rattled on the casket lid. Hospital friends, not family members, filled in the grave (suicide is, after all, a curse, and the family did not want to be affected by it), and I shared in that part of the mourning.

Just after we buried Onyango, Wafula came up to Jan and me. It was hot; there were no trees to stand under next to the fresh mound of earth over Onyango's body. It was the first time we had seen Wafula since Onyango's death. He told us, "I've been trying to avoid him since I heard that he died…Sometimes I feel like—did I let him down? He came to me for money, I didn't have much money, I gave him a little." We talked it through, sharing stories, wondering what it all meant. And then he told us something that stuck with me: "I think he didn't remember he was not alone. There were other people around. Once you think you are alone in the wilderness…Ah…." And again: "He forgot at one moment that he was not alone. He thought he was alone…."

It was a silhouette, an outline, of a dazzling truth that Onyango was momentarily blinded to by his troubles. *No one*, Wafula was saying, is alone—a truth that Africa still remembers in crowded buses and streets packed with people walking, walking and laughing together, while we in the developed West watch this truth slip away. We know it has to be true, this business of not being alone, and we try to hold on to it in our religions and our "friends" on Facebook and our support groups and our counseling… and all of these attempts are just more evidence that community is slipping away, and we are more and more alone—alone in our cars in a traffic jam, alone playing solitaire with a computer.

Onyango forgot; he was buried, wrapped in a white cloth, in a casket with a window in it. Wafula told us what he forgot, and in the process reminded me that I want to be buried naked.

*

All this, for me, is global health: friendship, sharing stories, working together, mourning, listening, and learning. There are no statistics in these stories.

2. Stuck in Global Health

I ADMIT IT: I'm stuck in global health—or at least my version of it. My version of global health is living where I work, not just visiting; my version is working for the health systems that are here, not introducing new ones. My version is at least as much about Wafula and Onyango as mosquito net programs and community surveys.

But it's not just me who is stuck. If major global health conferences are any indication, all of global health is stuck. Though I rarely attend them, I do get the itch every five to ten years: How is this field changing? What are the current trends? And mostly, what have I been missing? In May 2002, I attended the Global Health Council Annual Conference in Washington, DC, expecting to be brought up to date on the latest ideas from academic and government centers. I assumed that after 16 years "in the bush" I would be out of date, and was looking forward to being challenged. Instead I found people talking about the same kinds of programs they had been discussing 20 years before—and it seemed stale. Yet global health has not always been stuck.

My introduction to global health—it was then called international health—was at a MAP International conference and seminar in 1984. MAP, a global Christian health and relief organization, was a strong supporter of the kind of primary health care promoted in Almaty (formerly Alma-Ata), Kazakhstan, in 1978 (the Alma-Ata Declaration came out of that year's International Conference on Primary Health Care), and was introducing these concepts to people with careers in curative missionary medicine. It was exciting: clinical and public health people were talking with each other, exploring the possibility that rural villagers knew what their health needs were, and that we technical people should listen to them. Their communities, we were taught, should be the hub of any health and development activities; those activities would be most effective when they were "community-based."

To be sure, there was another approach still very much alive in international health, the "vertical" programs. In contrast to "horizontal" primary care programs, the vertical disease-specific programs were often "donor driven" and run by outsiders. These programs had some remarkable successes, such as smallpox eradication in the late 1970s; and some equally striking failures, such as malaria eradication in the 1960s. What made the mid-1980s such an exciting time for international health is that there was an active debate between the "PHC people" and the more traditional public health and clinical people.

By the 1990s, a new element had entered the conversation. In 1993 the National Council for International Health published *Global Learning for Health*, an eclectic collection of experiences and thoughts about how we can "bring international health back home." International health workers' experiences in innovative health programs in the Third World began to highlight the deficiencies in Western health care systems. These workers—perhaps having learned to listen from their community-based orientation—realized that approaches they were using overseas might work equally well in the "developed" West.

Admittedly, this idea of bringing home approaches that were learned "over there" has not caught on very well—though oral rehydration therapy has become the standard of care for diarrhea in US hospitals, and some communities have parish nursing programs that utilize volunteers similar to village health workers. But again, the importance of the ideas behind *Global Learning for Health* is that some people were reflecting on their work in light of what they came back home to, and there was the possibility of a debate between the people who had learned from international health and those who were still trying only to teach it.

With this promising background of listening in local communities, learning there, and bringing what we learned back home, I assumed (or at least hoped) that by 2002 there would be a new "global health": having considered the possibility that some communities may know what they need, and having realized that some of the ways "they" do things may be appropriate even for us, we can truly function as an interrelated global village. "Globalization" is the byword—the National Council for International Health changed its name to the Global Health Council. Now we can all, representatives from poor and rich countries alike, sit together at some global table and discuss as equals how to approach global health. That, at least, is the theory. My attendance at the 2002 Global Health Council Annual Conference, however, gave me a different picture.

My first impression of the conference was that I was hearing nothing really new. There were new technologies, new statistics, and new jargon, but these were all buttressing old approaches to global health problems. Old approaches are not bad per se; but after having been in the debates about top-down vs. bottom-up approaches, and after being convinced that we do need to listen closely to the people we are serving, I was surprised to find very little of this kind of conversation. I heard the results of innumerable studies, and the humanitarian pronouncements of many important people. And at the end, I heard pieces of a passionate debate—but even that debate seemed to miss something. So I went back to my notes to try and understand better what was bothering me.

- At a panel discussion titled "Maternal Mortality: A Human Rights Perspective," one presenter spoke of the need for safe abortions and post-abortion care. I commented that very few, if any, of the maternal deaths I had seen in 15 years had been related to abortions, either spontaneous or induced. The response was a statistic: 13 percent of maternal deaths worldwide are due to complications of abortion (meaning 87 percent were other complications of pregnancy). Yet of the 20 or so conference exhibitors dealing with family planning or women's health, I could find only 2 mentioning emergency obstetric care in their abstract. The emphases of our women's health programs didn't seem aimed at the main causes of death.

- There were a few places where Africans did question our assumptions—but very quietly, "in between the lines." At the launching of the African Council for Sustainable Health Development, one African health official was asked, "Why do all Africans say they are helpless? Why don't you do a better job coordinating donors?" His response was eloquent: "You cannot coordinate donors when you have your own vision." Do we realize the strain we put on African health systems when there are so many of us to coordinate? Do we spend any time listening to what that African vision is?

- And at the panel on "Tuberculosis and AIDS: The Critical but Ignored Linkage," the African presenter was Dr. Francis Omaswa from the Ugandan

Ministry of Health. He addressed his given topic well—and then, just before sitting down, said, "Our number one killer still remains malaria." We could have a statistical debate, but malaria still remains foremost in the minds of many Africans. Yet of all the conference panels and roundtables, 21 were on HIV/AIDS and only 4 were on malaria; and there were 10 booths in the exhibition hall dealing wholly or partly with AIDS, but none dedicated solely to malaria. Have we listened to Africa's priorities?

- Finally, I heard quoted yet again this proverb: give a man fish, and he will eat today; teach him how to fish, and he will eat every day. The proverb does address the "relief to development" question—but are we still assuming the fellow doesn't know how to fish? Since this is a global village, perhaps he has no fish because his river is polluted from other "development" efforts; perhaps he has fish to sell, but no market. The metaphor still works, as long as we remember that we are part of his economy, not just his savior.

- I did not hear the controversy around Thabo Mbeki[1] mentioned at any of the discussions on AIDS I attended, unless I raised it. Yet he was an important voice in the AIDS debate in Africa, and his views deserved to be examined, even if we didn't agree with them. The press had crucified him—but we, at this prestigious international health meeting, had done worse: we ignored him. Do we think the Western approach to AIDS is really completely appropriate in Africa? The one passionate debate at the end of the conference was about whether we work *with* drug companies to get antiretrovirals into Africa, or instead pressure the companies to lower their prices and in the meantime find generic drugs made in other countries. Yet the assumption on both sides was that antiretrovirals must be a cornerstone of AIDS care in Africa. A larger question, according to Mbeki, is the validity of that assumption—but it's not a question we asked.

- We heard a presentation by Edward Green at the pre-conference retreat of Christian Connections for International Health. He presented the findings of his research into why the incidence of AIDS is falling in Uganda, suggesting that a main reason for the decline is changes in sexual practices, not condom use. However, he had difficulty publishing his findings, one journal even telling him that his work was "dangerous" because people might stop using condoms as a result. He was listening to what the people of Uganda had been saying—and listening to his own findings—but the academic community didn't want to hear it.

In reviewing these reasons for my discomfort at the Global Health Council Annual Conference, I found a single theme running through all of them: are we listening? Community-based health care taught us that we should listen to poor people in the village—but that is a long, difficult process. It is no surprise that I heard once in a workshop in East Africa that as we facilitate development discussions in villages, sometimes we need to "facipulate": appear to facilitate, but really manipulate. Have we done the same thing with African nongovernmental organizations and ministries of health? Why are we so sure of our own agendas? One discussant in a maternal mortality workshop was concerned that as conservative anti-abortion policies in Washington influence funding for women's health care, the programs would become "donor driven"—seemingly unaware that her own pro-abortion programs were equally donor driven.

And what has happened to "global learning for health"? The ultimate result of listening to people is learning from them: we let what they tell us influence us and the way we function at home. True globalization means that we need to learn as much as teach, and receive as much as give; true globalization means we no longer control the agenda of how this happens. But I don't hear this need to listen and learn being articulated any more.

It seems instead that we think we know what the world needs. We speak a new "global" language, but often only dress up old neocolonial ideas with new technologies. In our shrinking world, we feel more intensely the weight of the world's disease burden, and declare without irony (as the conference program cover did) "when it comes to global health, there is no *them*, only *us*"—never realizing the double meaning of the phrase. The intention, of course, is to affirm a global interconnected "us," but the conference instead seemed to affirm a Western "us" trying to help a poor "them"—a "them" whose agenda seems not to exist.

Is it too late to start listening again?

*

Perhaps it is. In March 2015 I tried again to update myself—this time at the annual meeting of the Consortium of Universities for Global Health in Boston. To me, it seemed that global health was really losing its way. Or, possibly, it was simply becoming up-to-date, in sync with the latest advances of biomedicine and public health. In either case, it appeared that listening was no longer necessary in global health, that global health answers would be coming from well-conducted studies, from applications of the latest technology, but certainly not from the people being served.

For me, the best part of the conference by far was the student essay contest. The students were alive, fresh, honest, passionate; their stories raw and full of wonder, fear, anger, pity, and compassion. One student was robbed; another had her first experience watching children die; a third described mapping health facilities in a Haitian village that an earthquake leveled four months later.

In comparison, the rest of the presentations were careful, plodding, and self-assured. Like all good science, they were accurate, considering all possible variables, cautiously hopeful based on the evidence. They were about "platforms," "systems," "value chains," and "apps"; about capacity, scale-up, determinants, and assessment. Politics and culture were factored in, but only as "context." As usual, these scientific presentations decided what the question was, and then proceeded to thoroughly answer the question they just asked. But was it the right question?

To me, what was missing was the connection between the students' experiences and the academic answers.

Would it be possible to have a conference where the student essays were first, were in fact the introductory plenary? Students, as the main drivers of university global health programs, deserve a larger role than just an essay contest. Why are they studying global health? What do they want? Perhaps we could begin with their experiences, their impressions, their questions. The entire conference could be an ongoing dialogue, or dance, or sometimes even duel, between raw experience and careful science.

Both are necessary. Student interest is only one driver of global health growth; the other is, of course, careful science and the technological solutions it produces. These solutions from the industry, together with government desire for global health security, provide the technology, and the necessary funds, for the massive growth of global health.[2]

A conference that seeks to be a conscious live dialogue between those with fresh experience of the problems and those actively involved in seeking responses would itself be a unique contribution to this still burgeoning field of global health. And such a dialogue could prepare the way for the far more fundamental dialogue that still needs to happen: between global health scholars and activists in the West and those in the receiving countries.

Low- and middle-income country scholars know where the money, the technical expertise, and the high-paying jobs are; they increasingly know how to access these resources. But what do they really want? What are their visions for global health? Opening the essay contest to narrative essays by citizens of middle- and low-income countries would be a way to begin hearing voices we are not used to.

But this was not the conference I experienced in 2002, or in 2015.

3. "The Global Community Knows What Works"

IN JULY 2013 Mark Herzog, an undergraduate student from Duke University, stayed with us for a month while participating in a summer research project with one of his professors. As he was leaving Kenya, he requested to interview me by email—for one of his courses on global health, he had to prepare a portfolio that included an essay, a bibliography, a book review, and an interview. His topic involved improving maternal and child health in rural Kenya.

I found him very refreshing, first of all because of his ingenuousness. In November he wrote to me to introduce his topic, with his assumption drawn, I assume, from the global health courses he had been taking. "The global community knows," he wrote, "what medical interventions work to prevent maternal and child mortality, but the larger issue at hand is figuring how to bring these interventions to scale within specific contexts." His question to me was "about what allows a program to fit a local context—or even if you agree/disagree with the whole premise of my portfolio."

I initially chose to deal directly with his premise: "It is commonly suggested," I responded, "that 'the global community knows what medical interventions work to prevent maternal and child mortality' and that the big issue is appropriate applications of these interventions, given local contexts and cultures, etc. I partly agree; that is, some interventions have statistically significant 'evidence,' confirming their effectiveness—but of course, as you say, any project must be 'anchored in the local context.'

"However, I take issue with the primary assumption. First, we call it 'the global community,' but the assumptions of that community and the science underlying it are very Western. The global community, and specifically 'Global Health,' are NOT culture free, no matter how many people from developing countries sit on its policy-making boards, etc. Global health is a Western project, with motivations and ideas rooted in Western educational and political institutions. Consequently, saying 'the global community knows...' is a euphemism for 'the west knows....' That same community is the one that tests those known interventions for statistically significant effectiveness—and this 'evidence' is heavily dependent on who asks the question, and how the question is asked.

"Therefore, when we assume that these 'known' interventions simply need appropriate 'bringing to scale' 'in the local context,' we are assuming that the interventions themselves (and the science that developed them) are culture free—which they are not. My own thought is that the interventions themselves, and not just their local application, need to be developed in the local (or perhaps national) context."

I then went on to suggest several authors who underline how the socio-politico-economic context influences how we develop interventions, suggesting especially these two:

- John Farley, *Bilharzia: A History of Imperial Tropical Medicine* (Cambridge University, 1991), especially Chapter 2 "1898: A Declaration of War" (pp. 13–30) and Chapter 17 "Conclusion: The Imperial Triad", especially pp. 291–293

- Randall Packard, *The Making of a Tropical Disease: A Short History of Malaria* (Johns Hopkins, 2007), especially Chapter 5, "The Making of a Vector-Borne Disease" (pp. 111–149)

I then added this: "In both the Packard book (p. 136) and the Farley book (p. 173), they talk of a 'more expansive approach' (Packard) or 'social views' (Farley) which were present in the 1920s and '30s. 'But,' Packard adds, 'this vision did not survive the interwar period.' The big question is whether *any* global health approach today has rediscovered these 'more expansive approaches' of the social medicine that Packard and Farley say did not survive the interwar '20s to '30s."

Mark read everything I suggested, and less than a week later we began by email the following interview:

Mark Herzog: In our earlier exchanges, you pushed back on my assumption that the global community knows what works but still hasn't figured out how to apply this knowledge to a local context. I would like you to expand on that comment in this interview. To begin with: many of the readings you suggested to me make the point that given certain factors at the time, health research in tropical areas was pushed early on to a focus on biometrics (looking solely at the disease) even though early work highlighted the socioeconomic factors at play. Do you think this bias for biometrics is at play when organizations like WHO or UNICEF say that the global community knows what interventions work? Is it that the international community has hyper-focused on the medical problems while ignoring the larger factors at play?

Dr. Downing: Yes. But remember that those larger factors go beyond just the identifiable "socioeconomic." There are cultural, religious, ethnic, political, etc. etc. etc. factors. Some fundamental issues to consider are: Who is in control? Who is setting the agenda? Where is the money coming from? Where are the ideas coming from? These are all really the same question.

Mark: Do you think the focus on biometrics is leading to a failure in applying these valid interventions to local contexts and achieving results (i.e., is the problem that we haven't really figured out the socioeconomic factors and that until we do, health outcomes will remain poor)?

Dr. Downing: Partly yes—but even when we do figure out the socioeconomic AND CULTURAL factors, we don't focus on them. This is partly because a) they are so big and hard to change, b) we are medical people, not economists and development workers, and c) the interventions themselves were built on Western assumptions and not developed in local contexts. And all of this comes about because our interventions are much more often in vertical rather than in horizontal programs.

Mark: Is there a lack of resources and research in developing approaches to tackle these socioeconomic factors at play?

Dr. Downing: Yes…but even if Bill Gates was primarily funding socioeconomic research, I'd still be skeptical. The direction of research is very much determined by the funder. There is an African funder willing to give a million dollar prize to the best African leader each year, yet half the time the award is not given because they can't find anyone worthwhile. So part of funding is in knowing what NOT to fund.

Mark: One of the points I have wanted to explore in my research is the argument that many global health interventions are being invested in without having first established empirical evidence to support effectiveness in the local context. Would you agree with this argument given your on-the-ground experience?

Dr. Downing: Maybe…but there is a problem here. Your assumption seems to be that health improves as a result of the right collection of evidence-based interventions.

In fact, staying healthy is not rocket science, and the wisdom about it is very old. Example: sterile technique does not need to be re-proven. Why then don't hospital workers use it? Maybe there are not enough of them, and morale is poor. But why? They have insufficient supplies and supervision. But why? Playing the "but why" game keeps pushing us back toward socioeconomic, political, and cultural factors, NOT back to biometrics.

Mark: But can't evidence-based interventions be focused on which approach works best within a given set of larger socioeconomic, political, and cultural factors?

Dr. Downing: Sure. Given that in the current climate, answers and approaches seem to originate in the West, and we in the West seem to be the ones who have tasked ourselves with bringing them to Africa. A sort of contemporary White Man's Burden.

Mark: This past summer the President of Kenya declared all maternal health services free. From your experience in the field, how has this worked out so far?

Dr. Downing: The hospital (Webuye) IS doing more deliveries, somewhat, but will that make a difference in maternal and infant mortality? For that question we would of course need biometrics. But we are still seeing far too many maternal deaths. Without changing the nature, content, and quality of the free maternal services, there's unlikely to be a change in mortalities. I think I mentioned to you that 75 percent of women around Webuye deliver at home, and that distance doesn't matter until she lives as close as two km from the hospital. There's something else going on that needs to be addressed—but finding out that 'something' will involve qualitative socio-economic-cultural research, not biometrics.

Mark: Do you think that the decision to have free maternal health services was one where little evidence was gathered prior to its implementation to support its ability to address maternal and child health concerns?

Dr. Downing: It was likely purely a political decision, like handing out cash, designed to garner (i.e., buy) votes.

Mark: Do you think this is a pattern in strategies targeting maternal and child health in Kenya or is this just an isolated occurrence?

Dr. Downing: I sense (and have observed) that strategies undertaken generally follow funding, and funding is often "global," which means agendas are global—which means they are not local. The key issue is not evidence or its lack; the key issue is whose agenda is being followed? And that goes back to funding.

Mark: So whose agenda is driving policies relating to primary care in Webuye District? Don't practitioners have some level of control over what policies get put into place?

Dr. Downing: It seems to be that practitioners have

virtually no control of what is put in place. In the new devolved Kenya environment, control moves from the national level to the counties (with politicians on either level calling the shots). This is a matter of great concern right now, with a possible health worker strike looming next week. Watch the news. It might not happen, but something's got to give. Health care now in the government system is terrible and getting worse.

Mark: Is a lack of empirical evidence for strategies in the local context holding back improvements in health outcomes in rural Kenya?

Dr. Downing: Probably not—see all the above.

Mark: Earlier you stated that there's a lack of understanding of the larger factors. So isn't it a problem that no policies have evidence for their effectiveness in getting mothers into the clinic?

Dr. Downing: Sure.

Mark: Or in the case above, you stated that the President made a political decision to make maternal and child health free. Isn't that a problem if a policy decision as big as free maternal services is made without any evidence to show that it will help improve maternal mortality?

Dr. Downing: Absolutely. My problem is not with evidence per se. It is needed. My issues are about who asks the questions and how are they asked. "Evidence" is determined by how we pose the question, and we outsiders will likely pose questions differently than locals.

Mark: Many countries have used the idea of "task shifting" to utilize local resources and build a health system that incorporates lay health workers at the community level of care. Some of these countries have achieved remarkable health improvements and pointed toward their community health workers as the keys to success. Kenya has rolled out a similar community health strategy. Do you think there are issues preventing the community health worker program from achieving similar success?

Dr. Downing: Even in the '80s, community health worker programs sounded wonderful, but the actual successes were few and far between. Then they mostly died in the '90s and '00s, upstaged by war and AIDS and a relief paradigm. In 2008, the 30th anniversary of the Alma-Ata Declaration [the first international declaration calling for the improvement of primary health care globally], we started hearing about community health workers again—but no one seemed to be addressing the reason the programs failed: who was going to continue paying them?

Mark: Do you feel that the problems are because of an inability to apply this strategy to a Kenyan context?

Dr. Downing: No. See above.

Mark: Well, before you said that no one has addressed the reasons for why they failed. Doesn't that mean that no one has answered how to make this work in a context?

Dr. Downing: Well, again, the community health worker programs that came out of the Alma-Ata era were created at an international table, not a local one. Community health worker approaches were based on the barefoot doctors of China and similar strategies elsewhere. My view is that we DO need to reinvent the wheel everywhere because the terrain everywhere is different. Sand requires different sorts of wheels than pavement. Water requires floating boats, not wheels, etc.

Mark: You mentioned earlier that you think interventions need to originate from the local context. What do you think are some barriers to the development and scaling of local ideas in rural Kenya?

Dr. Downing: I think some interventions developed locally might stand a better chance of "working." But think about it: "going to scale" with a locally developed intervention is an oxymoron.

Mark: If the interventions originate from the local setting, does this mean that they will be more likely to succeed and improve the targeted health outcomes for the local setting?

Dr. Downing: Having an intervention originate in the local setting is no guarantee of success; it is not a "formula" for "doing it right." There is no formula. The best approach is to come and live in a specific location. LIVE there, not just visit with a specific time frame and goal, and see what you learn. At the end of it all you'll be so much wiser, certainly more cynical, with possibly no idea of what should happen to "fix things."

4. Global Health in History

WHAT IS REFRESHING about Randall Packard's new book, *A History of Global Health: Interventions into the Lives of Other Peoples,*[1] is that there is a clear theme running throughout the book, and it is developed remarkably free of social science jargon and is therefore readable. The theme is that working for global health means addressing the social determinants of illness and reinforcing basic health services. The readability makes this theme readily accessible to global health practitioners and activists.

Early in the book, in his Introduction to Part II, he writes: "...the 1930s raised the possibility of significant new approaches to international health, yet these changes remained more in the realm of vision and rhetoric than in actual achievements. In the end, international health interventions retained a faith in scientific solutions, a limited understanding and valuation of local cultures, and an inability or unwillingness to address the structural conditions that underlay patterns of sickness and ill health around the globe." This is a concise summary of his theme.

It is unfortunately a story not limited to the 1930s. The League of Nations Health Organization promoted the broader vision of health between the World Wars, a vision which never really took root in Europe's African and Asian colonies. Then after World War II, the new World Health Organization tried to resurrect the broader vision, but it was soon overshadowed by the focused attempt to eradicate malaria.

In the wake its failure, WHO returned to the broader vision of health, this time advocating Health for All by the Year 2000 at the Alma-Ata International Conference on Primary Health Care in 1978. But again, within only two years, the focus narrowed again, this time to "Selective Primary Care."

The vision for a broader understanding of health never dies, but it never thrives either. The seduction of efficient and effective medical technologies—magic bullets used in vertical programs—repeatedly overwhelms the less exciting longer term work of addressing social determinants of disease and building primary medical care.

However, the problem with efficient and effective medical technologies in global health is more than simply overshadowing work arising from broader social approaches. Packard subtly but incisively uses the letter "s" to expose another danger: global health not only intervenes for good or bad in the lives of people, but—according to his subtitle—into the lives of *other peoples*. That is, as he writes in the Introduction to Part III, global health programs historically "were designed by experts who met in cities in Europe and the United States to discuss and make plans for improving the health of peoples living in Africa, Asia, and Latin America. They also shared a confidence in the superiority of Western knowledge and a disregard both for the ideas and practices of those for whom the campaigns were created and for the ability of targeted populations to meet their own health needs." This was the early 1950s.

There is the same sentiment in Packard's title for Part V: "Controlling the World's Populations"—not just the numbers, he seems to be saying, but the people themselves. He is writing here not of colonial-era programs, but of the 1960s, 1970s, and 1980s.

Now in this era of Global Health we think that we are no longer colonial, that discussion and decisions are made at some global table attended by representatives from the entire globe. That table is there, but it's usually located in Europe or the United States, and the people around it are all educated according to the same Western-defined paradigms. Packard in 2016 could write that we—we decision-makers at that global health table—are still intervening in the lives of other peoples, and we are still trying to control the world's populations.

Unless, of course, we no longer think in terms of "other peoples" and "world populations." Perhaps cultural differences have been overplayed. We now view ourselves as just one global village. As the Global Health Council declared in 2002, "When it comes to global health, there is no *them*, only *us*."

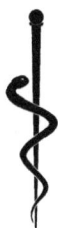

PART II:
AIDS

5. African Perspectives on AIDS

IN LATE 2003, shortly after she graduated from Boston University, my daughter Elizabeth and I made a trip to Africa. She had grown up with us in East Africa, and it was her first trip back since graduating from high school in Kenya four years earlier. My wife and I, after 16 years of medical work in Sudan, Tanzania, and Kenya, had returned to the USA in 2001—but we were failing re-entry. Africa seemed so much more, well, sane. Elizabeth and I were traveling to several countries, talking with as many people as we could—scholars, medical workers, friends made over 16 years—about how they viewed AIDS. I did not intend this to be formal research; I simply wanted to know if my hunch—that many Africans saw AIDS differently than it was being portrayed in the Western media—was true.

By this time, there were already several published reflections by African scholars on the African AIDS epidemic. While African scientists were often part of the biomedical search for effective ways to diagnose and treat the disease, African theologians and philosophers were more interested in how people were confronting this new disease, and how the Western approaches fit in a traditional African worldview. Western scientists, because of their vast infrastructure and experience, usually led the biomedical search; but it was African theologians more than Western social scientists who first probed the relationship between the biomedical approaches and how they were being received by people "on the ground."

As we traveled throughout eastern and southern Africa, talking to people "on the ground," Elizabeth jotted down these words from several of these people: "The press promotes a Western view." "The whole of Africa is in waiting until the answer comes from the West—and this mindset damages the African view of life." "They (in the West) have to understand the African mind." "Enough with Western answers." Put slightly more gently: "The West has some very good AIDS programs. But they are not always suitable for us. You may give me a pen when I want a pencil." And finally: "What if you asked us what we have? Why don't you build on what we know?"

I was reassured that the perspectives I had been reading from African theologians were reflected in the doubts and suspicions that we heard as we traveled. But it is difficult to summarize African perspectives in a single sentence, and partly because of this, most of us don't know what they are.

We should. Two-thirds of the world's AIDS burden is in Africa. A careful review of African writings reveals that Africans and Westerners do not always view the world with the same questions, concerns, and emphases. Before suggesting—and funding—programs to control AIDS in Africa, we need to be aware of how Africans understand their own epidemic. A good starting place is the writings of three African priests.

In 1992, Fr. Laurenti Magesa published *AIDS and Survival in Africa: A Tentative Reflection*.[1] Fr. Magesa is a Catholic priest and moral theologian, sometimes serving as a parish priest in Tanzanian villages, sometimes teaching in African or US universities.

He suggested three ways to understand AIDS in Africa—three "cosmologies." The first is the traditional one, where people function in a world of magic, taboo, and ritual. Problems in society develop when people "go against the demands of God as entrusted to the ancestors." I took a class with Fr. Magesa in 1998 in Nairobi. One of the students was researching AIDS on an island in Lake Victoria, and told us that the elders on the island believed exactly that: the AIDS epidemic there stemmed from ignoring the traditions of the ancestors.

While this view still clearly influences how people behave, Magesa said it was "inadequate from the contemporary standpoint…There can be no going back completely to that cosmological view." The second cosmology Fr. Magesa described is one that sees AIDS as "directly linked to sexual activity," but with people responding in a "confused" or "muddled" way. "In response to the threat of certain death caused by the disease, [their] behavior is not appropriate; it indicates nonchalance or even helplessness." It was this cosmology, "the confused view," that Fr. Magesa saw as predominating in Africa 25 years ago.

The third cosmology is the modern view, which sees AIDS simply as a disease linked to sexual activity, with the appropriate response being to limit sexual partners. In 1992 Fr. Magesa doubted that it was the predominant cosmology of most Africans. The number of AIDS cases was rising across the continent; with most people, the direct link between AIDS and sex, and the response to limit sexual activity, had clearly not yet happened.

And today? In 2013 Magesa gave us an update.[2] Today, he says, for Africans who have AIDS, "his or her sexual behavior is seen as the proximate and apparent reason for it, because educational efforts by governments and non-governmental organizations have impressed on people that HIV is transmitted mostly through sexual activity." So have they moved to the third cosmology? Not really. "The general judgment is that 'the power of witchcraft' or 'my bad behavior' toward some 'unknown power' is the ultimate cause of the affliction." Indeed, advertisements for traditional healers are as common in Nairobi as political posters, and are often placed side by side.

"In the current context," Magesa concludes, "where everyone is talking about the world as a global village, it is important to undertake an exploration into the particularities of the indigenous worldview of Africa."

*

Another African theologian who has written about AIDS is Fr. Benezet Bujo, a Congolese Catholic priest who has taught in African universities and is now teaching in Switzerland. In 1993 he published *The Importance of the Community for Ethical Action: The Example of AIDS.*[3]

For Fr. Bujo, community is foundational in an understanding of African cosmology. "The individual knows him or herself to be immersed in the community to such an extent that personality can develop only in and through it." Consequently, "because no clan member can live in unrelatedness, in cases of misfortune the cause is looked for within the community itself. According to African wisdom, a disease is always an indication that something in human relations is wrong." Later in the chapter, Fr. Bujo makes it clear that since AIDS is an international disease, it is reasonable to apply these principles internationally: "The problem of this disease is not an individual question alone, but possibly first of all a structural one." The community here is the entire world, and the disordered structures Fr. Bujo sees are unjust economic policies established by the northern countries, poverty, Third World debt, etc.

Naturally, "the reformation of our society is a task which cannot be mastered by the individual alone." Yet "in the discussion concerning AIDS, one often gets the impression that prevention of this epidemic is possible if the individual behaves more carefully." Fr. Bujo shows the inadequacy of an individual behavior-change approach: "'If an information campaign is satisfied with advertising condoms, without exposing the deeper causes and ignoring the ethical questions, then one is merely treating the symptoms.' Advertising condoms rather promotes the consumer mentality, reducing sexuality to a commodity…Only an ethical conviction is able to fight this consumer mentality efficiently and to restore sexuality its dignity…'Neither purely technical advice (use condoms, prevent AIDS!) nor moral admonitions (remain faithful!) are sufficient to control the disease. The prevention and stopping of AIDS does not depend solely on the individual but on the quality of our institutions, changes in culture, economy and politics as well.'"

Note carefully: Fr. Bujo is not against condoms because the church requires him to be. In fact, neither he nor Fr. Magesa rules out the use of condoms. He is, rather, cautioning against individual approaches to a disease that has communal causes. He is concerned about "condomization" and its effects on Africa. Fr. Bujo puts it this way: "From an African perspective, it is to be stated that an indiscriminate distribution of condoms ultimately wipes out African culture." He is arguing here as an African, not a priest. In fact, mentioning aspects of African tradition which "prepare for sexual self-discipline," he says, "colonial policy and European Christianity have already destroyed this cultural background…If the industrialized nations wish to help Africa, they should offer their support in such a way that the African people can recover their spiritual and moral immunity, which cannot be underestimated even if it does not offer or replace a technical solution for AIDS."

Ultimately, this loss of African culture hurts not only Africa but the entire world community. "The African community understands itself as a healing community," but this self-understanding is under threat. When Western medicine was brought to Africa by the colonists, it "was never integrated into people's consciousness; [rather] colonial systems destroyed the African medical tradition, which could no longer be effectively applied. For even if the Western type of medicine proved to be more efficient in many cases, the holistic approach to medicine was lost, since the modern method of treatment looked at the person merely from the viewpoint of 'repairing' one's organs."

*

The third African priest is Fr. Emmanuel Katongole, a Ugandan who is now on the faculty of Notre Dame University in the United States. His contribution is the paper "AIDS, Ethics and Society in Africa: Exploring the Limits of an Ethics of Suspicion," which he presented at a conference at Uganda Martyrs University in 2000.[4]

He begins with the assumption that Western approaches are now preeminent in the fight against AIDS, and asks how these approaches have affected Africa: "As we make particular decisions and choices, what sort of people are we becoming?"

He suggests that many Western views of Africa and its people contain misleading and racist attitudes, with the result that the objects of these views—first African scholars and intellectuals, but eventually all Africans—become suspicious of the West. He sees this suspicion increasing as a result of the AIDS epidemic and the West's narrow approach to it, which "narrowly focuses on 'viral infection' and overlooks the wider economic and political and general health conditions in Africa."

Though "we [may] need a certain measure of suspicion as part of the practical wisdom of everyday life and survival," says Fr. Katongole, becoming suspicious has a cost. Africans have not only become suspicious of the West, he says, but they have also been told by the Western approach to AIDS to become suspicious of each other.

> I remember in the early '80s when, at least in Uganda, billboards warning against the spread of HIV infection carried the picture of what was obviously a married couple with their three young children and bore the caption: "Love Faithfully to Avoid AIDS." This recommendation was soon replaced by the Uganda AIDS

Commission with what was seen to be a more potent picture: two young lovers in embrace, with the caption: "Love Carefully." What the Uganda AIDS Commission might not have realized, but what in fact it was confirming was the realization that with AIDS even lovers cannot (or is it, should not) trust each other fully (love faithfully), but must learn the art of loving "carefully," that is, suspiciously. Apparently it did not take a long time to realize that such "careful" love involves regarding the partner as potential danger from which one had to "protect" oneself. Thus, by mid '90s the captions had changed again, this time from "Love Carefully" to "Use a Condom to Avoid AIDS."

The West may have long ago adopted this mutual suspicion, but it is new to Africa. This "radical suspicion generated by AIDS gnaws at the very core of our self-understanding, and thus threatens the basic trust on which our individual and societal existence is based," the priest notes.

Instead of addressing how Africans can rebuild trust, the West has promoted condoms. One brand, provided by a US-based nongovernmental organization through social marketing, is even called Trust. This process of sidestepping the fundamental issues Fr. Katongole calls "condomization": "The issue of course is not whether condoms do or do not protect against the spread of AIDS...The issue is about the sort of culture which 'condomization' promotes, and the sort of people we become as a result." Condomization becomes a "metaphor for the incursion of postmodern culture in Africa."

Fr. Katongole, as an African, describes three fundamental problems with that incursion. Condoms are disposable, like so many other aspects of Western culture. But condomization "is not just about the convenience of disposable condoms, but more importantly it is about the popularization of a certain form of sexual activity, i.e., one detached from any serious attachment or stable commitment. In other words, condomization encourages one to view sex and one's sex partner(s) as essentially disposable, while at the same time parading such lack of attachment as a high mark of freedom and accomplishment."

This "freedom" is the second problem with condomization. Using a condom seems to confer immediate freedom—but, of course, "freedom does not come naturally, but is a result of *training* into the relevant virtues of chastity, fidelity and self-control." That, at least, is the teaching of church and tribal traditions. Without this training, these "free" people become "free-floating individuals who easily become prey to their own whimsical needs and choices."

These whimsical choices Fr. Katongole calls "nihilistic playfulness," the third problem with the incursion of postmodern culture into Africa. This sounds a lot like the confused or muddled cosmology that Magesa wrote about. When people begin to adopt this postmodern worldview, Katongole says, "we lose not only the possibility of locating ourselves within any meaningful material economic practices and history, but even more crucially, we become increasingly prey to the manipulations and misrepresentations of the media and market forces... It may not be a long shot to see a connection between this form of nihilistic playfulness and the various forms of desperate violence with many countries in Africa. Such violence may be just an indication that the extreme form of cynicism, namely fatalism, is, for many Africans, just around the corner."

*

These views, though presented here in an academic form, are broadly reflective of views I have heard during 15 years of medical mission work in Africa. The questions for these scholars, and for most Africans, are not focused on the microbe, or even how to introduce and fund antiretroviral drug programs. They focus on the overall cultural approach to health and disease. Their concern is not whether or not an individual uses a condom, but rather what is ignored when condoms become the essence of prevention. These people, the ones most affected by this epidemic, have a much broader view than we do. Why don't we listen to them?

6. Listening to Mbeki

IN JULY OF 2000, South Africa was host to the 13th International AIDS Conference—the first to be held in Africa. A slogan at that conference was "Break the Silence," both the silence within Africa about addressing the problem, and the silence in the world community about the scale of Africa's crisis. The silence was broken, and the world became more aware of Africa's AIDS disaster.[1]

A month or two previously, the President of South Africa, Thabo Mbeki, convened a panel of scientists to consider why the human immunodeficiency virus seemed to be acting so differently in Africa compared to the West; a minority of those scientists doubted that HIV caused AIDS. Mbeki also was not enthusiastic about government support of antiviral drugs given to HIV-positive pregnant women to prevent transmission to the fetus; he was concerned about their toxicity. These positions earned him scorn from the media, disgust from many AIDS activists, and accusations that he was denying the scope of the AIDS problem in his country. In other words, that he was not part of the UN program to "break the silence."

The degree of scorn in the media is notable. *The Guardian Weekly*, for example, began their coverage with a July 6 article entitled "Scientists denounce Mbeki's 'Aids error,'" followed the next week by a front-page article:

"HIV judge berates Mbeki for Aids confusion." The next week it was "Mandela unites Africa in battle against HIV"—interpreting Mandela's support of new drug treatments as a "coded message to…Mbeki" not to delay their introduction into South Africa. On August 24 there was an article entitled "Mbeki faces court battle on Aids drug," which included a reference to Mbeki "letting babies die." By September 28, *The Guardian Weekly* quoted several South African leaders opposed to Mbeki's position in "Friends turn on Mandela's faltering heir."

It wasn't just the press. In those days, whenever I would mention to a fellow doctor that the press seemed to be crucifying Mbeki, the response was usually "And so they should!" before I had a chance to finish what I was saying. The assumptions seemed to be that a) the HIV cause of AIDS is proven, b) it is important to affirm this in the fight against AIDS, c) anyone who doesn't is in denial, or just stupid, and d) when drugs are available for treatment or prevention, they should be made available and used. Period. Mbeki was questioning all of those assumptions. The responses I saw to this questioning were not simple disagreement, and certainly not analysis of why he was questioning, but scorn, disgust, and ridicule.

Should we question scientific dogma? I used to believe that peptic ulcers were not an infectious disease. I believed this because I was taught it by scientists who had investigated more deeply that I had. I changed my beliefs about peptic ulcers because some scientists kept an open mind, were willing to question dogma, and did further studies, and found *H. pylori*.

Mbeki felt we should question scientific dogma: "I am amazed at how many people, who claim to be scientists, are determined that scientific discourse and inquiry should cease because 'most of the world' is of one mind."[2] Most of the world thought peptic ulcers were not infectious, but scientific inquiry fortunately did not cease. Mbeki was only asking that scientific inquiry not cease for AIDS; if only in the name of true "scientific discourse and inquiry," his maverick position on AIDS deserved to be considered seriously, not ridiculed and scorned.

Mbeki was not alone. There was then in Africa a "loose confederacy of what some have termed as 'AIDS dissidents'" who "agree on one umbrella question: Are we satisfied—or to what extent are we satisfied—with the answers which the scientific establishment has offered regarding HIV/AIDS medical theory and development?"[3] One letter to the editor in *The Guardian Weekly* suggested that people read Mbeki's speeches in context, quoted a bit of one not otherwise referred to in the *Guardian* articles, and then said, "Anyone who has visited southern Africa's rural communities will be painfully aware that the solutions and programmes that work in London, Paris, Frankfurt, and New York will not work there. The media is doing Mr. Mbeki, and the search for an effective response to the Aids tragedy in Africa, a great injustice by insinuating that, by asking questions rather than regurgitating the 'truth' as seen from the developed world's perspective, he may be doing international efforts a disservice."[4]

That was only one letter, short and untitled. The news media has focused mostly on the questioning of HIV as the cause of AIDS, the one part of the dissidents' position which makes them look foolish in the eyes of the majority of scientists. The above quote of the "umbrella question," which shows the breadth and intelligence of the dissident position, was not in the mainstream press, but in a small bulletin published in Kenya. The real news story was that Africa was beginning to think about its own response to AIDS, and that story has been ignored by the international news media.

*

What did Mbeki really say? When he convened the scientific panel, it comprised a handful of dissident scientists (about 10) to discuss issues concerning AIDS with a larger number of conventional scientists (about 20). In May 2000, he introduced his concerns to the panel this way: "What we knew was that there is a virus, HIV. The virus causes AIDS."[5] He then asked the scientists to consider why that virus seemed to be acting so differently in Africa compared to the West. The media decided he believed what the dissident scientists did, and accused him of denying the link between HIV and AIDS. So in an interview two weeks later on US public television, he was asked where he stood on the relationship between HIV and AIDS. He said, "I don't know where these reports come from, that we're taking a position saying there's no connection…between HIV and AIDS. I never said it."[6]

What he did say a few months later in another interview was this: "If the scientists…say this virus is part of the variety of things from which people acquire immune deficiency, I have no problem with that." But that wasn't all: "Once you say immune deficiency is acquired from that virus, your response will be antiviral drugs. But if you accept that there can be a variety of reasons, including poverty and the many diseases that afflict Africans, then you can have a more comprehensive treatment response."[7] Once again: no denial of the role of the virus, but a plea for a broader approach than simply antiretroviral drugs.

And then, echoing the belief in an African cosmology that we noted above with Fr. Benezet Bujo, Mbeki said this: "[A] simple superimposition of Western experience on African reality would be absurd and illogical…I am convinced that our urgent task is to respond to the specific threat that faces us as Africans. We will not eschew this obligation in favor of the comfort of the recitation of a catechism that may very well be a correct response to the specific manifestations of AIDS in the West. We will not, ourselves, condemn our own people to death by giving up the search for specific and targeted responses to the specifically African incidence of HIV-AIDS."[8]

When antiretroviral drugs became the standard of care in the West, activists in South Africa demanded the South African government supply them free in all government hospitals. The drugs then were very expensive; their side effects, or toxicities, were well known. Considering the expense and toxicities, Mbeki's government decided to proceed cautiously with a plan to introduce them in hospitals, eventually in late 2003 presenting a comprehensive plan, of which antiretrovirals were one part. In retrospect, it may look like he proceeded too slowly.

It may also be that he was exactly right in proceeding cautiously. As important as these drugs are, we cannot afford to sweep all of the questions about them under the rug—questions about resistance developing and financial sustainability and the need to take the drugs for the rest of one's life and the lack of infrastructure to make them available. Success rates with the tuberculosis cure—a much shorter and simpler treatment course—made a good comparison. David Serwadda, a Ugandan AIDS researcher at Makerere University in Kampala, noted that HIV treatment "can't be any easier than tuberculosis, and we have 35% failure with TB." Even if "antiretrovirals were $1 a day, it wouldn't make much difference."[9] At the time, experience in Europe and the USA showed that

HIV-positive people took antiretroviral drugs only 50 to 80 percent of the time—and the golden number to prevent resistance is closer to 95 percent. Mbeki was right to think very carefully before suggesting that antiretrovirals are in any way an "answer" to AIDS in a continent where the medical infrastructure was, and still is, one of the least developed in the world.

This was 17 years ago. Now, using billions of donated dollars, Africa has extensive AIDS treatment programs, with drug adherence rates sometime better than those in the West. By the time those programs started, new AIDS infections had already started falling, and beginning around 2005 AIDS-related deaths also began falling. Likewise, mother-to-child transmission rates started falling around 2005, and continue to fall. It started to look like Mbeki and other critics had it wrong.

But that very success helped to mute the truth in what Mbeki was saying, to mask other approaches to the epidemic, to ignore the problems that will arise when funding runs out. As I wrote this, Donald Trump was about to become the 45th president of the United States. In preparation, his team "questioned the President's Emergency Program for AIDS Relief (PEPFAR), a programme that reaches nearly 11.5 million people with life-saving anti-retroviral treatment and has provided more than 11.7 million voluntary medical male circumcision procedures in Africa. The Trump team asked: 'Is PEPFAR worth the massive investment when there are so many security concerns in Africa? Is PEPFAR becoming a massive, international entitlement program?'"[10]

If donor money ceases, the massive antiretroviral programs may become a house of cards, and hopeful statistics will crash. Will we then realize that responses to this epidemic must come, at least in part, from within? Will we then start to listen to Mbeki?

7. Why Is It So Difficult for the West to Hear African Voices?

THERE IS PLENTY of room for debate about antiretroviral drug policy—but is there any room for debate about whether or not Mbeki denied the link between HIV and AIDS, as is still being reported? And since Mbeki's statements made 17 years ago are so clear, why then does the world still know him as the African president who denied the link between HIV and AIDS? We could blame sloppy reporting—or we could blame Mbeki himself, since some of his comments clearly deemphasized HIV as the sole cause of immunodeficiency. But neither explanation is satisfactory. There are plenty of excellent reporters in the media who could easily have found and reported the many statements Mbeki made affirming the link between HIV and AIDS. And Mbeki's comments about HIV not being the sole cause are not really unorthodox: many infections require co-factors. Why then was the South African AIDS story misreported?

We can begin to glimpse an answer when we consider how the rest of Africa heard Mbeki.[1] While the Western press in general vilified him, the African press felt he was on the right track. Where Western activists were angry with him, African scholars felt he was opening a discussion about how AIDS thrives in the context of African poverty, a contention they felt was obvious. Mbeki, as an African leader, dared to have an opinion about a matter that Western scientists felt they were experts in—and his opinion differed from theirs. It's not that he denied the human immunodeficiency virus, but he did proclaim that focusing on it alone—as with condoms to prevent it and drugs to control it—was an inadequate response to AIDS. Were the Western opinion leaders—scientists and the press—offended that an African dared to have a different opinion? Possibly, but they could get over that.

The problem is not just with the media and activists. In the preface to a recent book on AIDS in Africa and the Caribbean, the editors dealt with their lack of inclusion of African voices this way: "The editors are very aware of a major lack in this volume. We do not intend to marginalize or silence the voices of Africans and persons from the Caribbean, either researchers or AIDS victims. We are very conscious that research in Uganda, for example, could not have been done by the anthropologists and historian whose work you will be reading in this volume, were it not for Ugandans' willingness to share their knowledge and views. The two articles by David Serwadda, the clinician who first diagnosed Slim in 1982, are taken by Bond and Vincent as benchmarks in the history of the AIDS epidemic in Uganda."[2]

At first, this seems to be a simple humble recognition

of the value of African voices—except that instead of being an introduction to these voices, it is an excuse for not including them. Bond and Vincent apparently do a good enough job in telling us what Serwadda's contribution was. We never see it or any other African contribution directly. It would have been better to not mention the "major lack in this volume" at all, rather than to point it out and then do nothing about it—effectively marginalizing and silencing the African voices that are not in fact included.

It's a perennial problem. In 1990 several African scholars published *Beyond Hunger in Africa*,[3] the results of a 1987 exercise by those scholars to articulate alternative visions for Africa's future. The conventional wisdom then was that Africa was a continent in crisis because of famine; today the crisis is AIDS. The sentiments of the introductory chapter, written in the context of hunger, could apply equally to AIDS. Consider these excerpts:

> Perhaps the most tragic aspect of this situation is that the debate about Africa's future is dominated by the international community. Those who are farthest removed from African realities—who do not feel the pinch or who need not take responsibility—are the pacesetters. In fact, even more than in the past, the prevailing notion is that Africa cannot move ahead without the aid of the international community...As the 'crippled' region of

the world, Africa is largely treated in a paternalistic fashion...In brief, Africa today suffers in particular because of the following three shortcomings:

- The image of Africa is one-sided
- Africa's own voice is ignored
- Africa's domestic capacity is neglected

Some Western scholars agree. Paula Treichler, in *How to Have Theory in an Epidemic*,[4] says "deeply entrenched institutional agendas and cultural precedents in the First World prevent us from hearing the story of AIDS in the Third World as a complex narrative...In concrete terms, we need to forsake, at least part of the time, the coherent AIDS narrative of the Western professional and technological agencies and listen instead to multiple sources about and within the Third World."

Treichler is not alone. A more recent book, *HIV and AIDS in Africa: Beyond Epidemiology*,[5] recognizes the same problems. When "biomedical models remain dominant in generating understandings of AIDS in Africa," there is a "tendency in these studies to focus on sexual practices devoid of socioeconomic contexts," consequently ignoring "the social embeddedness of vulnerability." The larger question in *Beyond Epidemiology* is "how Africa as well as AIDS has come to be 'known,' what knowledge is privileged, and how it gets deployed. We are concerned, for example, that dominant interpretations of AIDS are aiding in the reproduction of problematic colonial and postcolonial African representations, practices, and social politics." The African scholars from *Beyond Hunger* in Africa would likely agree.

The authors of *Beyond Epidemiology* continue: "Perhaps the most visible example of what is at stake in conflicting interpretations of AIDS is still playing out in South Africa. South African President Thabo Mbeki's controversial stance on AIDS as a disease of poverty rather than an epidemic driven by HIV has caused profound consternation among international researchers as well as frustration among physicians and AIDS activists within South Africa (cf. Treatment Action Campaign at www.tac.za.org). While these concerns are more than understandable given Mbeki's refusal to provide antiretrovirals to affected populations, the incontrovertible dominance of biomedical models placing HIV front and center have silenced Mbeki's more insightful statements on poverty's role in creating AIDS in the South African context." That is a fair introduction to Mbeki—but in this 398-page book, it remains only an introduction. Mbeki is not mentioned again in the entire book. His "more insightful statements" remain "silenced." To be sure, there are other African voices in the book—but "the most visible example" is dropped. Why?

Why is it so difficult for the West to hear Mbeki and other African voices?

On one level, concerning Mbeki at least, the answer seems simple. We have seen how in 2000, Mbeki engaged in extended conversations with scientific "dissidents" from the West, some of whom deny that HIV causes the disease AIDS. Since the vast majority of those working with AIDS accept the link between HIV and AIDS—and since Mbeki was presumably guilty by association with these dissidents—the easiest approach was to ridicule Mbeki, and then dismiss him. This was the commonest response in both the media and among scholars, as shown by an example from a prominent medical journal.

The July 1, 2004, issue of *The New England Journal of Medicine* contained an article looking at AIDS in South Africa.[6] The author, Solomon Benatar from the University of Cape Town, said "The approach of the South African government to HIV and AIDS has been resoundingly criticized within the country and internationally. It has been a disappointment that a new, enlightened democratic government could so arrogantly deny the link between HIV infection and AIDS in the face of overwhelming evidence provided by the global scientific community… [T]he president, the minister of health, and others in the government have long publicly denied the link between HIV and AIDS…" Though this assertion has been stated innumerable times in the media, there is no basis for it. Mbeki never denied the link between HIV and AIDS.

But more than this, the footnote Benatar uses to

support his contention actually opens a door to some of the deeper issues of why we have trouble hearing black African voices. To Benatar, the important question was not Mbeki's contribution, but whether or not the dissident scientists were correct, and the footnoted article by the president of the South African Medical Research Council, M. W. Makgoba, indeed roundly criticized the dissidents.[7] However, Makgoba had far more to say in that article.

He began with a summary of what the current South African government "under President Thabo Mbeki" had done regarding AIDS, concluding that its "preventive and management programmes are the envy of the world," and lauding the "spirit of scientific independence within the broader framework of the African context, consciousness, conscience and social responsibility." Then, after his critique of the dissident scientists, he asked, "Why do the media of our country fail to highlight these positive initiatives and report accurately on the nature of this controversy?" He went on, "The media has also failed to see the big picture—the picture of an international holistic strategy that links the whole HIV/AIDS epidemic to national socio-economic and national development. The emphasis here is about solutions rather than causation." By highlighting "this holistic approach," which he attributed to the UN and other international agencies, he was pointing beyond simply settling the microbial etiology question. Having already declared his allegiance to the HIV-causes-AIDS position, his critique of the media was for being stuck on the dissident question, reporting it inaccurately, and failing to report the positive activities of the South African government. None of this made it to Benatar's *New England Journal of Medicine* article. Why?

Let's step back a minute and look at the elements of this story. The conventional perception is that Mbeki communicated with dissidents, therefore Mbeki was a dissident, therefore he should be exposed and countered. This view exists because the mainstream media—which saw some of Mbeki's speeches and interviews as ambiguous—presented it this way. Makgoba, as we saw, felt that the media failed to report accurately.

In addition, Mbeki's approach was not limited to the biomedical model in his analysis of AIDS, an approach he shared with Treichler and the authors of *Beyond Epidemiology*, as we saw above. However, the biomedical model remains dominant in the West. Scholars who quietly depart from it are tolerated; well-known politicians who depart from it and may be able to influence policy are not.

Taken together, then, we have a well-known politician who departs from narrow biomedical scientific hegemony and is reported inaccurately by the media. It's a ready-made tabloid story: dramatic, scandalous, exaggerated, and false. But why, then, were the writers and scholars of

Beyond Hunger in Africa excluded from consideration by those self-appointed pacesetters in conquering hunger in Africa? Why is it so difficult for the West to hear African voices like these?

The underlying questions here are questions of knowledge and power—questions openly debated in the academic world, but often invisible to the public. What is True and how we decide what's True—and who decides—are critical questions, but can seem obscure and arcane even to a concerned and literate public, and especially the part of that public who lean toward activism rather than philosophy. The discussions are, nonetheless, important. Let us listen to what two Africans say about why we have trouble hearing them; the first relates to power, the second to knowledge.

"'With AIDS we are seeing a replay of a dynamic which has occurred between the Third World, particularly Africa, and the West many times before,' says Nigerian Eddie Iroh, a senior international journalist and novelist. 'The Western media is bigger and better funded, and possesses superior communication technology, than the Third World, and so its voice is most often heard. This dominance makes it difficult for Africans to air their points of view, and especially to combat what many see as anti-African propaganda.'"[8] The point here is not whether or not the media is reporting accurately, but which media is doing the reporting. It is difficult to hear African voices simply because they are not as loud as the Western ones.

But, we may respond, facts are facts, regardless of who reports them. Yet even that defense carries an assumption that there is such a thing as a culture-free fact, and that the methods of science are value free. More and more voices are saying they are not. V. Y. Mudimbe, an African philosopher, commenting on how Westerners have viewed him and his continent, describes their "epistemological ethnocentrism; namely, the belief that scientifically there is nothing to be learned from 'them' unless it is already 'ours' or comes from 'us.'"[9] His concise sentence contains a profound point: how people from the West listen to voices from Africa is predetermined by what they already know. Our Western scientific paradigm inhibits us from hearing the knowledge born in other paradigms. It is difficult for the West to hear African voices because, to us, *there are no African voices* different from our own voice. The ultimate fate of epistemological ethnocentrism, or epistemological arrogance, is to be alone, unencumbered, and unaffected by other views, isolated from them so much that we don't realize they exist.

But they do exist. There are African voices, different from the voices that won't stop talking long enough to realize that there are other voices. Our first step must be to stop talking. And then listen, listen carefully.

8. Listening to Silences

UNFORTUNATELY, MBEKI NEVER got a chance to fully develop his views. The Western press was relentless, and the political cost in South Africa itself apparently was too high. After two years of struggle, Mbeki turned his attention to other matters. We never listened to what he was really saying about AIDS.

Following this silence, I asked Professor Emmanuel Katongole, the Ugandan priest, where I might have access to African voices as the antiretroviral programs were scaling up in Africa. Katongole answered, "You rightly note the silence of African debates on this issue. I personally am not surprised by the absence of African voices. After Durban 2000, and after Mbeki, that should not surprise you. Any views that African philosophers, physicians, theologians, ethicists might have had were buried within the Mbeki controversy. To me, Mbeki was the last African voice, and his dismissal was the official eulogy of any 'African' perspectives. Anyone who wishes to discover any African perspectives might have to do so by patiently learning the art of discerning the silences."[1] Katongole then went on to write a paper subtitled "Naming the Silences,"[2] which I will now draw from.

Before 2000, the AIDS epidemic in Africa was shrouded in silences: many African governments were silent about the extent of their epidemics, many African people were silent about their own infections, and the rest of the world was silent about Africa bearing the preponderance of AIDS internationally. Consequently in 2000 the XIII International AIDS Conference was held in Durban, South Africa (the "Durban 2000" Katongole referred to above), and the theme was "Breaking the Silence."

Many of the silences just noted were broken. Ironically, though, as these silences were being broken the resulting activity and noise effectively masked even deeper and more important silences. What are these deeper, more important silences the world must attend to as it grapples with AIDS? Professor Katongole and I discussed this together extensively; I will follow his outline in naming three silences of the modern approach to AIDS. We are silent about them not because they are secrets and we are trying to hide something. No, we are silent because they are assumptions, and sometimes we do not even notice them, let alone critique them.

A New Wall of Separation

The first observation Katongole makes is that when Western science discovered that the origin of AIDS is likely in Africa, this reinforced several old stereotypes of Africa: a dark, dangerous place inhabited by primitive, promiscuous people. We in the West are mostly silent about this stereotyping. Yet more than the stigma often discussed within Africa, Katongole was concerned that AIDS as Africa's own epidemic was increasing the stigma toward Africa from the rest of the world.

Prejudice against Africa was not new, but Katongole was pointing out that the power of science to "discover" and name AIDS created yet another reason to be suspicious of Africa. Even when the West decided to help—the massive 5-billion-dollar President's Emergency Program for AIDS Relief started by President Bush—Katongole saw this as a "merely humanitarian intervention," one that did not question the wall of separation between "those who live in an age of miraculous medicines and those who can only be the beneficiaries of the former's humanitarian largess." Miraculous medicines do not automatically bring people together; in fact, they may have the opposite effect of emphasizing our differences.

As an African priest-scholar, Katongole's concerns went beyond the medical treatment of a chronic infection. He was looking for caring communities of love and support, communities that could confront and dissolve the walls of separation between the infected and the uninfected, between providers of largess and recipients, between those who have and those who don't. Not surprisingly, he is drawn to the Apostle Paul's celebration of Christ's death and resurrection that broke down all walls of separation: "For he is our peace, who had made us both one, and has broken down the dividing wall of hostility…" (Ephesians 2:14).

Beyond Biological Individualism

One of the reasons biomedicine has been so successful is that it understands disease as located within bodies. Pathology is *biological* pathology; we direct medical interventions to people's bodies—and very often we see improvements. But, Katongole says, we are silent about the limitations of this approach, and the profound individualism inherent in it. African identity, he reminds us, always has a corporate element: "I am because we are; and since we are, therefore I am." As successful as an individual biomedical approach may be, it will always be incomplete. "Individuals," he writes about Africans, "could only be considered healthy if they belong to a healthy community."

This communal understanding prompts Katongole again to seek caring communities of love and support to complement individual biomedical treatments. This concept, we have just seen, is embedded in the best of African traditional culture. He also sees these communities in the biblical concept of *shalom*—meaning not just peace, but health, soundness, and well-being.

Yet, together with this affirmation of *shalom*, he expands on his critique of biomedical individualism. He quotes from Fee and Krieger, who point out that the biomedical model is "profoundly ahistorical" and "contains within itself a dichotomy between the biological individual and the social community, and then it ignores the latter...

Reflecting an ideological commitment to individualism, the only preventive actions seriously suggested are those that can be implemented by solo individuals…Intended or not, these attitudes implicitly accept social inequalities in health and fail to challenge the social production of disease."[3]

Katongole and Fee and Krieger are not alone in this critique. In Part I we saw that the theme running throughout Randall Packard's new book on global health in history is exactly the same. Any health intervention is incomplete unless it addresses the social determinants of health.

Obscuring the Whole Story

Still looking at this same problem of the narrow focus of biomedicine, Katongole asks us to consider disease in light of a major 19th century debate. Before Pasteur and Koch definitively worked out the germ theory of disease in the 1870s, academic thinking about disease causation was divided into two big ideas: miasma and contagion. According to miasma, disease resided in *places* that were unhealthy. It could have been the atmosphere there, the smells, the rotting vegetation, the filth. To prevent disease, people should avoid these places, or clean them up. Contagion, on the other hand, taught that disease resided in certain *people* who could pass the disease on to others near them. Preventing disease in this paradigm involved quarantining the people who had the disease until they were no longer infectious.

Not surprisingly, both methods—cleaning up places and quarantining people—worked to prevent some diseases. But when Koch and Pasteur found bacteria *in people* and were able to demonstrate those germs as the cause of their disease, it appeared that contagion had won. It was *germs*, they felt, not environment, that caused disease. The paradigm was set, and this narrow focus on germs eventually led to enormous success in controlling and killing germs through antisepsis and antibiotics.

Germs in people were not the whole story, though. Only 30 years after the proof of the "germ theory," Ronald Ross found malaria germs (parasites) in mosquitoes that lived in miasmic areas. Now the contagion vs. miasma debate was renewed using more scientific language. Ross advocated for the control of mosquitoes; Koch declared, "Treat the patient, not the mosquito"—and quinine very effectively treated the patient. Since then, it has been far easier to see the immediate success of treating patients than the more gradual results from cleaning the environment—and contagion, reborn as biological individualism, trumped miasma, reborn as environmental health.

This was the debate that Mbeki re-entered when he declared, "As I listened and heard the whole story told about our own country, it seemed to me that we could not blame everything on a single virus."[4] Mbeki never denied that HIV was involved in the causation of AIDS. Rather, he was emphatic that we needed to involve ourselves in the *whole story*: the same whole story that Katongole and *shalom* and Fee and Krieger talked about; the same whole story that Randall Packard's new book is telling us we should never forget.

One More Silence

Now listen to one more silence: how an African healer might see the world of science. These are the thoughts of Densu, the young healer in Ayi Kwei Armah's novel *The Healers*: he "saw a world in which some, a large number, had a prevalent disease. The disease was an urge to fragment everything. And the disease gave infinite satisfaction to the diseased, because it gave them control."[5] Listen too to his teacher Damfo: "...he who would be a healer must set great value on seeing truly, hearing truly, understanding truly, and acting truly...You see why healing can't be a popular vocation? The healer would rather see and hear and understand than have power over men. Most people would rather have power over men than see and hear."[6]

Science (including scientific healing) is successful precisely because it leads to power over the world and the people in it. But there is a caveat. A warrior tells Damfo, "I saw the weakness of the whites. It wasn't military at all. It was a weakness of the spirit, the soul. The whites are not on friendly terms with the surrounding universe.

Between them and the universe there is real hostility. Take the forest here. If they stay long in the forest, they die. Either they cut down the forest and kill it, or it kills them. They can't live with it."[7]

Though science is not the only way to understand the world and live in it, it is the way that those who would control AIDS use to bring about that control. The deeper silence of the scientists is in failing to openly admit that their way is not the only way to understand either AIDS or the world. Power over nature, even nature harmful to humans, is not the only way to avoid the harm. If the forest is dangerous, is cutting down the forest the only way to avoid the danger? Apparently people who have always lived in the forest don't think so.

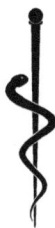

PART III:
FAMILY MEDICINE

9. What Is Family Medicine in Africa?

FOR THE LAST dozen years, my wife and I have been faculty members at a Kenyan university, helping to develop Kenya's first family medicine training program. Though we had worked for nearly 20 years in East Africa prior to starting, we were certainly not Kenyans. Yet we were hired directly by the university, not seconded from a nongovernmental organization or American university. And since my work, at least, was primarily administrative, that meant I had to deal *as a recipient* with donors and other expatriate do-gooders. Some of them initially viewed me as an ally, because we shared Western training and culture. But part of my task was to evaluate how their contributions would fit with what we had begun, and to coordinate them. If I suggested their contribution did not immediately fit, their view of me rapidly changed from an ally to a local person they needed to patronize. Sometimes I didn't even need to disagree.

Early on in my time as department head, one of the do-gooders, a PhD expert from Europe, in Kenya less than 24 hours, brought me to the local club, bought me a Coke, and began grilling me: "What is family medicine in Kenya?" We were in the first year of training, struggling to implement a curriculum which was intentionally written in vague and general language to allow us to deal with his important question.

"Well…I don't know. You see, in the US where I trained…"

"I don't care about the US!" he interrupted. "What about here? What is family medicine here?"

"What I meant to say was that the general practice I've been doing here for the last 20 years is quite different from the family medicine I learned in the US…."

But the expert was not interested in what I learned in the USA, or what I had done for the last 20 years. Or what Kenya needed. I clearly had inadequate answers for his questions. Simply to take the heat off myself, I asked him if *he* knew what family medicine was in Kenya. He did, and he told me: a picture of family medicine much like that in his own country.

He saw family medicine as primarily caring for outpatients, those either with chronic diseases or "undifferentiated illness" where our job was to make a diagnosis. Those ill enough to need hospital care would be sent to the hospital for the specialists to care for.

Then I tried to explain (in those early years I was always trying to explain *some*thing): first contact primary medical care in Kenya was done mostly by nurses and clinical officers. People sick enough to need hospitalization were sent to general hospitals run mostly by medical officers with no training beyond internship; there were then few specialists. If we as postgraduate-trained family medicine doctors restricted ourselves to outpatient care, we would be referring the sickest patients we saw to be cared for by doctors with a lower level of training than ourselves.

But the European expert was not moved. "That," he shot back, "is not our problem. We need to practice family medicine. Let the government sort out what happens in the hospitals."

I remember being livid that he thought he knew what we needed after he had been in the country for less than 24 hours. Livid, but unable to show it, because I was now the recipient, and I was quickly learning that recipients are very careful about arguing, and never say no.

This story sets the scene for a dynamic very different from when I was trying to understand AIDS in Africa. For one thing, I was administering nothing then, only asking questions, listening, trying to understand. Now I was directing a program—and obviously should know what I was directing. With AIDS, there was a well-established literature that I could read; now the closest we had was extensive literature on primary health care in Africa—not exactly what we were teaching. With AIDS there was the public emotional story of Mbeki that I could engage with; now there was no public story as a sounding board for what we were doing. In other words, we were *importing* something new—and the medical school dean understandably told me: "You are the technical experts; you know your product. We will help you administratively, but you are the ones who know what family medicine is."

Now if we were bringing in the first surgery program, that approach would make sense: surgery is the same worldwide, since anatomy is the same worldwide. But family medicine deals with families, with culture, and ultimately with the set of diseases most commonly found in those settings—and we were certainly not experts in that culture and those diseases. But—the response comes quickly from those advocates of a universal family medicine—surely the *principles* are the same: comprehensiveness, continuity, context-based bio-psycho-social care.

The principles do seem universal for the communities where the principles were developed: industrialized communities where chronic diseases make up a high proportion of the disease burden. Imposing them on a community where acute infectious diseases, maternal and perinatal conditions, and undernutrition are common makes less sense. We could affirm the notion of a generalist physician, but felt that the notion of family physician as developed in the West could not be simply lifted from abroad and taught without modification.

I was caught. I was in the position to bring something in, but I didn't feel it was appropriate. My first step was to try to redo the product, make it more compatible. So I did what I always do when I want to figure something out. I wrote.

I began to reflect on family medicine in Africa long before I started working in it. When I heard in the 1990s that some mission hospitals wanted to introduce family medicine training, I could not see the connection between the way I was trained and the health problems I was confronting in Tanzanian and Kenyan mission hospitals. But I did see the need for doctors to have postgraduate training beyond internship. When those missionaries working together with Moi University invited me to share some thoughts at a planning meeting in 2000 convened to advance the development of family medicine training in Kenya, I agreed.

The source I relied on to raise questions and suggest some alternatives was Maurice King's 1966 book *Medical Care in Developing Countries.*[1] I had long been drawn to King's analysis because it seemed so logical to me. He had developed 12 axioms as guiding principles to follow in designing medical care in countries that had only recently been released from colonialism. The subtitle of his book underlined his major premise: "A Primer on the Medicine of Poverty."

By using some of those axioms, and comparing them with some of the accepted principles of family medicine such as comprehensiveness, continuity, and bio-psycho-social care, I was suggesting that we needed other models for family medicine than the one designed mostly for chronic disease care in industrialized countries. But, in retrospect, it was not helpful to underline poverty as the "main feature determining" the "pattern of care" that King wrote about.[2] Being aware of poverty is important in designing any health-care system, but it is not Kenya's only reality today—and Kenyans understandably feel insulted when outsiders assume it is. Kenya still has marked poverty: about one half of its people live on less than 2 dollars a day. But there is also a great deal of wealth in Kenya, meaning that the more important dynamic today is inequity. And because there is wealth in Kenya, both monetary and intellectual, why are we outsiders still trying to come up with the models to solve Kenya's problems?

But I was, then—though I should have known better. Several years before this I wrote a book on my experiences in "poverty medicine," two-thirds of which took place in Africa. I sent the manuscript to Fr. Laurenti Magesa, the Tanzanian priest referred to in Chapter 5, and he offered some very kind comments. Near the end of his comments, he wrote, "I kept asking myself as I read: How can medicine incorporate itself into the African understanding of life as a unity of mind and heart, mind and body, individual person and society, humanity and the cosmos? What elements in the African experience of disease can help make medicine not only a curing experience but also a healing one? Can medicine in Africa cease to be looked at as 'poverty medicine,' with the unintended negative connotations of that phrase, and just be seen as medicine in Africa?" Why, he was asking, of all the defining characteristics of medicine, should poverty be the defining characteristic in Africa?

10. Magesa's Challenge

MY NEXT ATTEMPT to figure things out was, in retrospect, a direct response to Magesa's challenge. It was late 2004; I was now working as a faculty member in family medicine at Moi University, and we were about to welcome the first set of trainees. I was finishing my manuscript on African understandings of AIDS, and wanted to extend this experience of listening to try and imagine African understandings of family medicine. I again read through the writings of several African philosophers and theologians, trying to articulate what might be the "African Roots of Family Medicine"—the title I was proposing for this as an inaugural lecture to launch the program.

I am quite relieved that I never delivered this lecture. Reading it now a decade later, I wonder what I really expected of doctors just beginning training in a new field. At best it is a record of my own convoluted view of the endeavor we were beginning, full of answers to questions no one was asking. At worst it was me trying to tell Africans who they were. It was inappropriate for new trainees.

Nevertheless, my never-delivered lecture was a part of my journey in trying to listen. I have extracted here several parts of that lecture that still seem relevant to me over a decade later. The rest—the embarrassing parts—I have left out.

*

General practice has been around as long as there have been doctors, and many involved in health care believe there is still a need for generalist primary care physicians. Family medicine, as a discipline, is much newer (only since 1969 in the USA), and carries with it not only the generalist "skills package," but also its own philosophical approach to healing. In the USA, this approach includes concepts such as continuity and comprehensiveness, and is focused on the outpatient treatment of acute and chronic diseases—and, increasingly, on preventive services. The approach was developed in response to specific needs in the USA, and in the West generally.

But we are in Africa. Family medicine training has begun in several African countries, and is about to begin in Kenya. The mostly unasked but critical question is: do we transplant Western family medicine to Kenya, or can it be reborn here? My bias is clear: since family medicine in the USA grew in response to specific needs there, we should not simply adopt that response, which is America's philosophical approach to healing. Family medicine needs to be reborn in Kenya.

I would like to begin by looking at the circumstances under which Western, scientific medicine arrived in Africa—both how it was introduced and how it was received.

Western medicine came to Africa as part of both the colonial and mission projects. Neither were primarily health projects, but both saw the developing 19th century medicine as part of the Western civilization that they assumed Africa needed. "Civilization and evangelization were complementary aspects of Christian mission," says Professor Jesse Mugambi. Consequently, neither the colonists nor the missionaries differentiated between the medicine they brought and the culture in which it developed. What happened with the mission project may be instructive regarding what happened to medicine. "To show that one was a Christian," Mugambi says, "one had to adopt the new way of life and thought, at least superficially…The Church demanded to isolate him from his primitive and heathen background, but his own conscience forbade him to do so. He was torn between two forces. Most Africans resolved the problem by living 'double lives'…This solution meant that in practice, moral issues could not be openly discussed at a depth which would reveal the tensions in which Africans were living."[1]

In other words, the Christian message came with Western "baggage," and the missionaries expected Africans to adopt the baggage along with the Gospel. While accepting the Gospel, Africans could not adopt the cultural baggage and were forced to live "double lives," assenting to the baggage in church, but not at home. Similarly, Western medicine came with Western baggage. People readily accepted the treatments (when they worked), but could not simultaneously reject their own traditional ways of healing, something the Western doctors kept hoping for. Africans were forced to live double lives with medicine as well as with the Gospel. "The missionaries could not feel and appreciate this agony, for they were not products of the culture to which African Christians belonged."[2] Missionaries had brought Jesus to Africa without realizing Africans already knew God. Likewise, doctors brought penicillin to Africa without realizing Africans already knew about healing.

Nearly half a century has gone by since colonialism officially ended, and now Africa has her own theologians and doctors. Or should we say that only 45 years have gone by since the colonists left, but missionaries and neo-colonialists still abound? In either case, many Africans still find themselves living double lives, caught between their indigenous understanding of the way the world functions and the seductive offerings of the West. Seductive, but not necessarily bad. Penicillin is seductive because it works. The problem comes when we assume penicillin will work for every disease. The problem also comes when we assume that because we have penicillin, we no longer need indigenous understandings of healing.

Before considering the contribution that family medicine can make to this dilemma, however, we must look at another project involved with medicine in Africa: primary health care. With the failure of the top-down public health projects of the colonial era, particularly malaria control, international policymakers proposed a new focus for health services, especially in developing countries. Primary health care of the 1970s and 1980s was intended to focus on first-contact and preventive services based in the communities in which the services were needed, not imposed by a colonial power. Primary health care depended on international *guidelines*, but the *control* of the services was supposed to be national, or even local. Primary health care also gave a role to Western medicine, but interestingly it was a subordinate, supportive role. Optimal health, said primary health care, depended on sanitation, nutrition, education, and *basic* treatments, often delivered by nurses or even village health workers. It was a system doctors should know about and support, but it was not built for them.

In villages, primary health care kept trying to ensure that its offerings were culturally appropriate. However, since it was an international project, not a specifically African project, there were places where the messages were foreign. Once again, though to a lesser extent than with colonial and mission projects, some people solved the problem by living double lives. "The African Christian continued to affirm whatever he was expected to affirm publicly, but in practice he did what was most practical to do in order to survive."[3] A similar dynamic occurred with primary health care "converts" in the 1970s and 1980s. African doctors responded in two opposite ways: they either became experts in the primary health care rhetoric, or they ignored the project altogether. Nevertheless, as with Christianity, much of what primary health care had to offer could be useful in Africa.

Now we are at the beginning of a new project, the introduction of family medicine to Kenya. As we begin, there may be some value in looking intentionally at how much of this project is foreign to Africa, and might result in family practitioners or their patients living double lives. At the same time, there may be parts of this project—as was the intent with primary health care—that could be rooted in African values. If we succeed in identifying and affirming these African roots, might it be possible for family medicine to avoid the "double lives syndrome"? Other medical specialties in Africa have not had the opportunity to do this as consciously as we can, because they see themselves to some extent as "culture free." Success in surgery, for example, does not depend on integrating with local diviners, but on a sterile environment, good technique, and a well-trained team. But at its best, family medicine is very conscious of culture, considering both the context in which disease occurs and also "reflecting the values of the society that it serves."[4] It gives us permission to ask where it—this family medicine project itself—comes from and whether or not it is consistent with who we know we are. In addition, family medicine has built into its very name a cultural agenda: the understanding of family. This is where we need to begin.

Professor Mugambi says that "the family is basic to all human society."[5] John Mbiti elaborates: "Each person in African traditional life lives in or as part of a family. The family is the most basic unit of life which represents in miniature the life of the entire people."[6] In the West, we need to be very intentional about this perspective and struggle to retain it. Modern scientific thinking pushes us in the opposite direction; it is very reductionistic and asks us to look intensely at smaller and smaller pieces to try to understand the whole. African thinking has never lost this larger perspective, that "the individual exists only because others exist." Mbiti calls this "a basic African view."[7] If this understanding of people in relationship is fundamentally African, then Africa provides a firmer foundation for family medicine than does Western society.

But we cannot stop there, with this vague affirmation of Africa's family-consciousness. We need to probe deeper, to see what this value means for African life, and what it might mean for family medicine. Benezet Bujo, the

Congolese philosopher, says that "because no clan member can live in unrelatedness, in cases of misfortune the cause is looked for within the community itself. According to African wisdom, a disease is always an indication that something in human relations is wrong."[8] On hearing this, the most scientific among us might protest. It is neither fair nor accurate, we might say, to blame an individual's hernia or malaria on the family or community. Families may bring stress and inherited disease, but not microbes or cancers. How can we who practice Western scientific medicine understand this deeply felt belief that "disease is always an indication that something in human relations is wrong"?

This is a difficult question, because it gets to the core of the problem of "double lives." Two completely different worldviews are colliding here. If we don't confront them, the "moral issues [involved cannot] be openly discussed at a depth which would reveal the tensions in which Africans were living," in Mugambi's words. On the other hand, if we allow a dialogue between the views, and maybe even reconciliation, we not only reduce the risk of double lives, but also enrich both the traditional African understanding as well as modern family medicine.

Considered carefully, the African view may not be as strange as it first seems to Westerners. Considering what might be wrong in family relationships does not usually prohibit Africans from eventually seeking help from biomedical practitioners. Africans do not mind undergoing therapies that deal with their symptoms; they simply feel that accepting medicine or surgery does not complete the therapy. It is good to rid themselves of the microbe or tumor, but they still need to find out why they got it in the first place.

Western thinking has a parallel view: good family practitioners realize that disease has causes far beyond microbes and genes. Habits (such as cigarette smoking) and practices (such as sleeping under mosquito nets) can greatly influence health, and these practices are learned from family members. Likewise, a strong individual immune system is dependent on good nutrition and peace of mind, both developed in the context of family relationships. In fact, it would make us better physicians if, as we dealt with the microbe or tumor, we would also be looking for why our patient got it in the first place.

Laurenti Magesa, the one whose challenge prompted me to listen to Africans, summarizes what must be at the core of any African-rooted approach to healing: "Besides the profound sense of God and the hereafter, [there is] the perception of life as the ultimate good and…community as the context of the possibility of human existence."9 This one sentence condenses the essence of African philosophy and provides a framework for building a truly African family medicine.

11. Family Medicine Research

FEW DOCTORS WERE really interested in "the essence of African philosophy" or "building a truly African family medicine." When Professor Chepkwony from the Religious Studies Department on the main campus would join me in medical ethics discussions with our trainees, we found first of all that much of this sort of material was obvious to the trainees; obvious, but not very relevant, they felt, to their study of medicine. And as time went on—and we got older and the trainees got younger—we sensed a move in them from "not very relevant" to "a waste of time." I had tried to take Magesa's challenge to young Kenyan doctors in training, but found that the conceptual gap between the traditional African worldview and their scientific training was too great. Or this more troubling thought: had I become the Westerner again lecturing Africans?

About this same time I became involved with a new networking group of family medicine training programs across Africa. One of the foundational tasks was to engage in research toward developing a definition of family medicine in Africa. It was exactly the question I had been asking for several years—and it was an opportunity to learn qualitative research techniques. I joined several experienced South African researchers, and together we started formally listening to what those interested in family medicine in Africa were saying.

Our first project[1] was to poll faculty members in African family medicine departments on what should be included in African family medicine curricula. It was our first experience together in structured listening: we listed the known characteristics of family medicine and asked them to evaluate how important each one was in their setting. We found broad agreement about core values, but the scope of practice was somewhat different in Africa: more inpatient care and surgery, less outpatient first-contact care.

Aware, however, that this project began with known (Western) characteristics of family medicine as the starting point, we were curious if there were other values and characteristics we were missing. In our second project,[2] we performed 16 in-depth interviews in 8 different African countries of generalist doctors who had been in practice for at least 5 years. Besides developing a picture of the benefits and constraints of general practice in Africa, we confirmed that the overall characteristics we had been assuming for family physicians—for example, attempting to view patients holistically—were reflected in our interviews with generalists.

Our third project[3] brought us directly from considering "what is family medicine" to all of the issues involved in establishing it in Africa. We interviewed 27 academic and government leaders from 9 different African countries, inquiring how they understood family medicine and its relevance to their settings. The consensus was a general recognition of the potential value of family medicine in Africa. However, the respondents were concerned because in most countries family medicine was not well known or poorly understood, and often lacked support from medical councils or even other medical specialties. Interviewees were attracted by the broad range of tasks family physicians would have, but saw the need for more clear articulation of their role within the existing health systems.

I personally was most interested in the concerns these leaders expressed. Qualitative research, I had learned, was not intended to prove as much as discover something. It was a formal, scientific way of listening. It was not only concerned about what the majority said, but what everyone said. Therefore the role of "outlier" responses was quite unique: they could of course be isolated, idiosyncratic views. But they could also be unique articulations of widely held feelings.

There were several bold outlier responses from this latter project that attracted my attention. I had been working for almost ten years to help get family medicine established in Kenya, hoping that it would soon take on "a life of its own." And when graduates were eventually posted (most by the government, as they were government employees on study leave) they were not posted as "family physicians"—no one knew what that meant. Instead, they ended up filling in where the need was—as pediatrician, or internist, or clinic and emergency doctor, or medical superintendent. Quality doctors continued to apply for training, but not in huge numbers. I was looking forward to hearing what academic and government leaders would say about this.

These are some of the warnings I found from the interviews, warnings that struck me as true:

Malawi: "…we don't have ways that would retain these doctors, having attained a specialist status, in the places where we want them to work…"

Rwanda: "…doctors don't want to live in places where they are not satisfied, like in remote areas where many hospitals are located…We send doctors in rural areas and after days they come back and set their private clinics and work for their own…"

"…but now to be like a surgeon or pediatrician, you know, you get more recognition in society…"

Kenya: "Family medicine practice requires a high level of integrity and a lot of commitment because indeed by any standards the family physician would work in a setup that perhaps very few would want to go and work under… because of the level of commitment and the integrity that is required of that officer…"

Uganda: "…family medicine has been going on for 20 years, but there are still very few family medicine practitioners…"

Nigeria: "…they are not playing as visible and important role as they should be…"

In other words:
- Doctors want status, and family medicine does not offer that.
- Family medicine often means remote rural practice, and few doctors will want to do that.
- Even in countries where family medicine had existed for 20 years (e.g., Uganda and Nigeria), it was still not well recognized.

When I listened to our research, it told me why I was, after ten years, still struggling to make progress.

*

In 2009, the networking group that was sponsoring the research held a major conference and invited people interested in family medicine from across the continent. They asked Professor Otsyula, my supervisor, to give a keynote speech. He was well respected because, as dean at our medical school, he welcomed and strongly supported family medicine training—despite being a cardiothoracic surgeon. They had good reason for selecting him.

His speech provided another exercise in

listening—literally. The sound system was not good, and Professor Otsyula read the speech rather than speaking extemporaneously. I was sitting near the back, and beside me was one of the European leaders of the networking group who—as I sat forward and strained to make sure I got every word—drifted off to sleep. The sections of Otsyula's speech that really woke me up seemed aimed at the European next to me, nodding off.

For example: "International declarations are nice statements made at international meetings which may or may not apply to the target. The recipients are often represented at the meetings by people who know better than argue in situations where they have already lost, or people who have no courage to say no."

Regarding dialogue on what family medicine is: "We appear to be making little progress. Several questions then arise. The first question is: who is discussing? The discussion is spearheaded by experts coming from outside the region, supported by few local people. The local people may be genuine in their quest for family medicine, or are they opportunists who see something to gain personally? The second question is: what is central—family medicine per se or the health of the people? The issue should be the health of the community, but too often one gets an impression that what matters to some people is to start family medicine in Africa. This may be doing a disservice to a good course and we run a risk of complete rejection."

Regarding why, despite increasing health budgets, African countries often see little improvement in health: "There are many reasons for this; among them is importation of inappropriate Western models and lack of appropriately qualified manpower. The Western models are built for upper-income groups in countries where there is sufficient manpower to meet the needs of the society. This would not be appropriate in countries where more than 50 percent of the population lives below the poverty line in underserved areas."

Professor Otsyula then made eight suggestions about moving forward with the regional dialogue on family medicine. These are the four suggestions that caught my attention:

1. "The curriculum must fulfill the standard content for family medicine described in the WONCA [World Organization of National Colleges, Academies and Academic Associations of General Practitioners/Family Physicians] guidebook, but in addition must reflect local needs and take into account the health-care delivery systems operational in the country."

2. "Whereas the doctors must be prepared to serve the underserved, an effort must be made not to portray family doctors as doctors for the poor, which would unnecessarily make the specialty carry the stigma of poverty."

3. "It will be necessary to get away from Western models."

4. "As this meeting works on the resolution for Africa, it should avoid the rhetoric of standard international resolutions. It should go out of its way to accommodate the recipient in a meaningful way."

None of the keynote speeches were included when the conference proceedings were eventually published, and Professor Otsyula's offering as a recipient was not accommodated in a meaningful way, and has never been published.

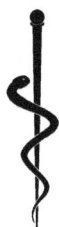

PART IV:
CHRISTIAN REFLECTIONS

12. The Christian Roots of Global Health

MEDICAL MISSIONARIES WERE the first global health workers in Africa; that alone is reason enough to look at global heath in the context of the faith that sent the early doctors from Europe and North America to Africa, often to die there. The common understanding is that they were risking their lives to spread Christianity by converting people, and that is partly true. But then why *medical* missionaries? Was this simply a spreading of the whole package of Western civilization, including the ineffective medicine of the day?

Maybe. But Didier Fassin sees another reason for their selfless activity, one that continues today in global health. Discussing contemporary humanitarianism, he writes: "The ethos from which it proceeds has its source in the Christian world."[1] Then, quoting Hanna Arendt, he explains further: "The reason why life...has remained the highest good of modern society" comes from "the fabric of a Christian society whose fundamental belief in the sacredness of life has survived."[2] In other words, the motivation driving the earliest global health workers, despite their proselytizing and spreading Western civilization, was at root their Christian belief that human life is sacred because God created and sustains it. And a sentiment derived from that belief survives even today in the humanitarian impulse which drives much of contemporary global health.

Partners in Health, a secular nongovernmental organization founded by Paul Farmer and his friends, is more explicit about this link between their activity and its source. Their mission statement begins "Our mission is to provide a preferential option for the poor in health care." The phrase "preferential option for the poor" originates in Catholic social teaching, and is a pivotal concept of liberation theology. Partners in Health continues: "At its root, our mission is both medical and moral. It is based on solidarity, rather than charity alone." The reference to "charity alone" here implies a narrow donating of goods or services, without asking why they are needed. On the other hand, solidarity assumes a relationship, walking with, accompanying those being served. And more than this, the accompanying inevitably leads to a concern for social justice—the "asking why."[3] This moral basis—the relationship and the work for social justice—are certainly consistent with, and even rooted in, the Christian world that Fassin recognized.

For Paul Farmer himself, the link with the Christian world is not merely a remote inspiration. His conversations with Fr. Gutierrez[4] reveal a close link between his approach in global health and the insights of liberation theology. The purpose of the recent Orbis book *In the Company of the Poor: Conversations with Dr. Paul Farmer and Fr. Gustavo Gutierrez* was to explore this link. In several places, the editors encourage Farmer to expand, aware that, as Gutierrez writes, "Dr. Farmer is a bit shy and reluctant to expound on theology and spirituality," yet recognizing that "his practice speaks very much to this matter."[5]

The editors of the book consequently asked Farmer to comment on a chapter in Gutierrez's *We Drink from Our Own Wells: The Spiritual Journey of a People* entitled "Conversion: A Requirement for Solidarity." Farmer admits that since he was not trained in theology, he decided to comment by drawing on fields in which he had been trained—medicine and anthropology. He then emphasizes the social and political conversions he sees as important in attaining social justice.[6]

Later, in a joint interview with Gutierrez, Farmer is asked where he finds hope as he works in "the darkest of places." He said that patients who get better give him hope. A "serious equity plan" gives him hope. "If you apply modern medicine justly with preferential options for the poor plus accompaniment, you have the most hopeful endeavor you can imagine."[7] So though Farmer does see a link between his faith and his activity, he apparently does not expect spirituality to *sustain* global health; his hope is in the medicine that makes people well and the resources that allow for an equity plan.

It seems that Farmer, as a Christian, draws inspiration from liberation theology—but he leaves the articulation of that inspiration to the theologians. Eleven years before Farmer was born, Jacques Ellul explained a dilemma in this model of theological discourse: "In reality, theologians today no longer have anything to say to the world...On the one side there is the pastor who does not understand the world's situation, and on the other there are the lay-people who go about carefully keeping their faith separate from their life." Gutierrez does have something to say to the world, but not specifically about global health. Farmer later openly admits that his spirituality plays a role in his work, but chooses not to discuss that role in detail.

Ellul continues: Christian intellectuals "necessarily have a particular function, in the world and in the church. They cannot avoid doing theology, because their vocation as intellectuals calls them to think out their faith. But they do not need to be specialists in theology...However, they do need to undertake a kind of practical theology... they have a very specific function...that no one else can do in their stead [and] a very specific mission toward the world."[8]

The next three chapters in this book are my attempts, undoubtedly flawed, to reflect theologically on what we do in global health. In each case, the reflection is rooted in an issue I have faced. These are examples; I hope they are consistent with the kind of "practical theology" that Ellul mentioned.

13. Justice and Listening

PAUL FARMER AND his colleagues call the first decade of this century the "golden age of global health"—and the stimulus for this golden age was AIDS and the world's response to it. "In the space of thirty years," they write, "scientists identified the pathogen and developed the necessary tools to turn what had been a death sentence into a manageable chronic disease." This—"modern medicine at its best"—was followed by massive funding for those tools to be applied where they were needed most: "an equity plan" that included funding for AIDS as well as malaria and tuberculosis. Science plus money precipitated the golden age.[1]

Equity, especially health equity, has to do with reducing barriers so that we approach equal opportunity for all; reducing inequities is a matter of human rights. How can we understand matters such as equity and human rights biblically?

As these concepts are related to justice, perhaps there is merit in looking at what justice involves from the first Servant Song in Isaiah 42. The task of the servant is justice, mentioned in verses 1, 3, and 4: "He will bring forth justice...he will not falter or be discouraged till he establishes justice on earth." But the methods—the core of the passage—are not what we expect: "He will not shout or cry out, or raise his voice in the streets. A bruised reed he will not break, and a smoldering wick he will not snuff out." Justice in this passage does not begin with "activism," with a political program like the Jubilee year, with advocacy as in "pleading for the widow," or even with a service intervention like feeding the poor. All of these are biblical ways to bring justice and enhance equity and human rights—but not first.

The beginning of justice, it seems, is quiet respect for those who have been trampled on, listening to their "agenda." The opening the eyes of the blind and freeing the captives from prison is just a few verses down, but the beginning of justice is sitting quietly in the presence of the bruised reeds and dimly burning wicks, making sure that what they have to offer is not broken or snuffed out.

We—the biomedical establishment of the West—have decided that AIDS is Africa's biggest medical problem, and that the centerpiece of our response should include antiretroviral drugs. Before the golden age began, it was clear that these drugs were too expensive for most Africans with AIDS, yet they were available for people in the West with AIDS. It appeared to be a clear human rights abuse—it was unjust—that those who needed the drugs most did not have access to them.

While denying antiretrovirals to Africa may be a human rights abuse, is it not also a human rights abuse to impose *our* understanding of Africa's biggest problems on them, to not seek out and listen to African perspectives on this disease? Does the world public health community know what the African debates are? Have they sought the opinions, not only of poor women dying from AIDS, but also of African researchers and scholars? Few in Africa would deny that AIDS is a major problem, but not all Africans feel it should upstage all other health problems. Clearly the poor women dying from AIDS are bruised reeds and dimly burning wicks in Africa—but does the world research community realize that African researchers and scholars are also bruised when their questions are ignored, and burn dimly when international research agendas and funding channel them into the Western debates?

Professor Otsyula's previously cited comment about "international declarations" refers to this dominance of Western voices in global health conversations: "International declarations are nice statements made at international meetings which may or may not apply to the target. The recipients are often represented at the meetings by people who know better than argue in situations where they have already lost, or people who have no courage to say no." Bruised reeds, smoldering wicks.

Our first task, then—as the chapters in Part II redundantly emphasized—is to listen. But we cannot listen if we do not know the language of those we have come to serve—not just the grammatical language, but the style of communication, the local idioms, the metaphors, the silences. Most African scholars, even those educated in the West, still have a mother tongue; they function very well in English, but the patterns of speech they heard before they could talk are imprinted on them, just as the patterns we Westerners learned at the breast (or the bottle) are imprinted on us. When we begin to engage in dialogue about "issues" as they were first articulated in Western languages, we need to remember that the conversation is far advanced before we ever start: we have already set the terms of debate. And when we do listen to African scholars, we mostly listen using European languages—meaning that what we hear has already been translated.

We need to learn to truly converse, in its literal meaning (*con* = with and *versare* = to turn); we need to dialogue *with turning* in our own position; we need to *turn with* those we are listening to. What we don't understand may be an opportunity to expand our own view of global health, to bring it closer to being truly global. And then, when we finally get around to offering what we have, we can offer it far more humbly, and listen very carefully to the response. And to discern the silences, because the silences may indicate disagreement.

This leaves us with a very practical question: does justice require global health workers to learn the language of the people they are working with? The answer goes directly to the heart of what global health is. If, as we discussed in Chapter 3, the global community knows what works, and the task of global health is to implement this locally, there is little need for language learning. Global health is then like international air travel: an Air France pilot talking with the control tower in Beijing uses English, and lands the plane successfully without knowing a word of Mandarin.

But the contention of this book is that global health is not like international air travel; that global health is relationship, which means listening. More than this, global health implies equity, or justice, and the beginning of justice is listening. Should we all, then, rush off to language school?

Language school is a good idea, as long as we understand what it means to really learn someone else's language. Ivan Illich is helpful here. Based on his experience learning Spanish as a parish priest in a Puerto Rican neighborhood of New York in the 1950s, and then teaching Spanish to potential missioners and development workers in Mexico in the 1960s and 1970s, he reflected on the importance of language in our relationship with the people we have come to serve. Some of his comments about American Catholic missioners learning Spanish 50 years ago are still relevant for global health workers today:

The first learning of a language must be more than the attempt at the acquisition of a skill, even more than the capacity to communicate…It can easily become a symbol of a man's willingness to become profoundly poor, to relinquish his own world of thoughts and associations and expressions 'as the best there is,' as the standard measure of fully developed thought. The acceptance of a local history and climate and socioeconomic structure can be more than the expression of a generosity which embraces physical discomfort for the sake of Christ. It is rather the expression of an eager willingness to become one with the missioner's new people. The acquiescence to foreign culture norms or behavior and taboos, besides being a necessary and utilitarian accommodation and a mark of delicacy and charitable toleration, can become an imitation of the Incarnation in a unique and typically missionary way.[2]

For Illich, language learning is an example of the "willingness to become profoundly poor," a quality he understands as foundational to working in another culture. That kind of poverty is equally necessary for work in global health: the ability to put aside, at least momentarily, all of my presuppositions and choose to actively listen. For Illich, this is following Christ's example in His Incarnation.

Illich knew also that when we learn a language, we

are in the position of accepting a gift from the people we have come to, and that language learning must always be receiving, not taking:

> If the missioner…attempts to conquer by his own power that which only others can bestow, then his existence begins to be threatened. The man who tries to buy the language like a suit, the man who tries to conquer the language through grammar so as to speak it 'better than the natives around here'…is a man who tries to rape the culture into which he is sent…He continues to preach and is ever more aware that he is not understood, because he says what he thinks and speaks in a foreign farce of his own language. He continues to 'do things for people' and considers them ungrateful because they understand that he does these things to bolster his own ego. His words become a mockery of a language.[3]

It is hard to imagine how we can truly listen if we have not received first from a people the gift of their language. Is language learning then necessary for global health? You decide.

14. Development in Babylon

IN THE SAME way that chronic disease care has become an unquestioned element of clinical medicine, so goal setting is now a standard element in public health. The UN is fond of developing these goals: Health for All by the Year 2000, the Millennium Development Goals, and now the Sustainable Development Goals.[1] The latter describes the world we all want: no poverty, zero hunger, good health for all, reduced inequalities, sustained economic growth, peace and justice. These goals are as obviously good as keeping someone alive through chronic disease care, and Christian health workers support them as much as anyone else.

We should look more closely. The world we long for, where there is no mourning or crying or pain or death, is a post-apocalyptic world, the world after the return of Christ. That world comes only after the fall of Babylon[2]—the biblical metaphor for all empires. The kings and merchants of today's Babylons have enough excess wealth to be able to imagine a world with no poverty or hunger or inequality, to even set sustainable goals to achieve those ends. But the biblical narrative does not see any Babylon and its kings and merchants achieving zero hunger and good health for all and an absence of the mourning that goes with death and disease. It sees rather the collapse of Babylon.

Nevertheless, the Bible is quite clear about hunger and poverty and peace and justice. From leaving the gleanings of the field for the poor and sojourner in Leviticus 19, through the multiple injunctions in Psalms and Proverbs about concern for the poor and Isaiah's blunt "seek justice, correct oppression, defend the fatherless, plead for the widow," to Jesus's spelling out what he had been doing—"the blind receive their sight, the lame walk, lepers are cleansed, and the deaf hear"—and James's exposure of the injustice of "the wages of the laborers who mowed your fields, which you have kept back by fraud," the biblical ideal looks a lot like the world of the Sustainable Development Goals.[3]

It is easy to understand, then, why a global health journal rooted in biblical thinking would develop a theme issue around "Sustainable Development and Human Flourishing."[4] Their initial argument in the call for papers was that the public sector was increasingly recognizing the role of faith-based nongovernmental organizations in achieving the Sustainable Development Goals, viewing religion as one of the social determinants of health. But religion in this sense is a sociological quality. Any religion offers this; there is nothing distinctly Christian about it. Our first task as Christians should be to critique the development goals themselves, and the means of arriving at them.

What is this development that is now so assumed that

we can remove the word "development" from Sustainable Development Goals and simply call them "global goals"?[5]

The appearance of this development coincided with the conclusion of World War II and the ending of the colonial period.[6] The "developed" world, the rich countries that had nearly destroyed each other for the second time in one generation, decided that the rest of the world needed developing. For the next half a century, they debated the nature of this development, a debate that took place in the context of the new Cold War. The Soviet Union and its allies believed that development would come about through central government planning, employing social-ist or communist principles. The West believed that the capitalist market alone was sufficient for development. Yet note that for both sides there was a fundamental agree-ment on two points: 1) the rest of the world—the "Third World"—needed "development," and 2) development meant *economic* development; all other aspects of national interest—culture, history, environment, religion—were secondary.

However, with the collapse of the Soviet Union, there is no longer a debate on *how* to arrive at this economic development. "Development" now has only one meaning and one method: free markets. And in order for market economies to function, they must grow.

Yet by the 1970s it was very clear that the earth and its people could not withstand unlimited industrial growth, which was tied to unlimited economic growth. Books with titles such as *Limits to Growth* and *Small is Beautiful* appeared; their titles speak for themselves. The development discussion was maturing, and Christian thinkers were at the core of this discussion. In 1964, Jacques Ellul's *The Technological Society* appeared in English.[7] Here he made clear that, despite economic differences between East and West, both were committed to technology as the means of "progress." Unfortunately, there are no built-in negative feedback mechanisms in the growth of technology. We have an imposed "technological imperative": what can be done will be done, and we call that "progress."

Building on the same Christian understanding,[8] Ivan Illich in 1980 defined "development" as "the transformation of subsistence-oriented cultures and their integration into the economic system." He was clear about the implications of this definition: "This expansion proceeds at the cost of all other traditional forms of exchange."[9] Illich made clear what was by now becoming obvious, that Third World development was only *economic* development, a development that progressively erased indigenous cultures.

In the first decade of post-colonial "development," Illich saw what was happening in Latin America. He could have been writing about Africa today: "Underdevelopment as a state of mind occurs when mass needs are converted to the demand for new brands of packaged solutions which are forever beyond the reach of the majority…The ruling groups in these countries build up services which have been designed for an affluent culture…Once the Third World has become a mass market for the goods, products, and processes which are designed by the rich for themselves, the discrepancy between demand for these Western artifacts and the supply will increase indefinitely…[ultimately] money is needed not for the uplift of the poor, but to protect the frail beachhead into the middle class that has been gained by the few converts who have benefited here or there by the American way of life."[10]

Then in 1989, when the communist vs. capitalist debate began to evaporate with the fall of the Berlin Wall, the nature of the economic system into which all subsistence-oriented cultures were integrated was no longer debatable. The only system left was the Market. The market, as we noted above, works by growing. Today, everything is growing, straining the ability of the earth to sustain that growth. And that growth increasingly benefits the very few. Five years ago, the world's richest 388 people controlled as much wealth as the poorest half of the world's population. When I wrote the first draft of this in early 2016, that "rich club" had shrunk to only 62.[11] One year later it was 8.[12]

In this bleak economic environment, how can Christians think about development? Perhaps it is not so important that we *as Christians* embrace the Sustainable

Development Goals. Our ultimate task is love, not statistical change. Of course, we can choose to work in projects that build systems and measure their output as data, if that is our occupation—but as Christians that is not the same as our *vocation*, our calling. When we love, statistics may not improve. And if statistics do improve as a result of our work, we should not kid ourselves into thinking that that is a true improvement needed in the world. We still live in Babylon.

The Sustainable Development Goals are short- and medium-term goals; they, and the measurement of them, are means to an end. Jacques Ellul frequently pointed out that in technological societies all of our activities have become means. We are so focused on techniques that we neglect true ends; our technological means have become our ends.[13] There is nothing wrong with measurable goals—which may be means to some greater end (such as human flourishing or human redemption)—except when those means become the ends in themselves. And they can easily become ends, because we can control means far better than ends. We can understand and engage with means, precisely because they are specific and measurable and achievable and all the rest. If we as Christians fully embrace the Sustainable Development Goals, we must never forget that they are only means. If we forget, these goals will be just as cruel a joke as Alma-Ata's "Health for All by the Year 2000."

15. Global Health: Is Suffering Necessary?

IN DECEMBER 2014, *Time* magazine chose "The Ebola Fighters" for its Person of the Year cover story. And while they wisely chose to highlight African as well as Western global health workers, most of whom did not get infected by the virus, it was three American medical missionaries who did get infected that made the story so compelling. Christian global health workers had suddenly become celebrities. But did they do anything special, anything uniquely Christian? Many who shared the Ebola fighters' honor were from humanitarian organizations such as the Red Cross associations and Médecins Sans Frontières, not Christian missions.

The motivational indistinctness in the Ebola fighters' story is worth pondering and provides a very contemporary example for us to ask: is there a distinctive Christian approach to global health, or do we simply draw from the myriad approaches already described, testing each piece for how well it reflects general Christian principles? Christian Ebola fighters had experiences very parallel to humanitarian fighters. Is Christian global health then simply a matter of finding the overlaps of global, health, and Christian in a Venn diagram?[1]

This seems to have been the approach since Christians

first became involved in global health over 200 years ago. Early medical missionaries, while often passionately evangelistic, built the medical side of their ministry squarely on the emerging secular biomedical paradigm.[2] The same is true today. In the 1970s, primary health care offered a much-needed critique to a purely biomedical model, a critique influenced by the Christian Medical Commission[3] and vigorously adopted by the Christian nongovernmental organization MAP International.[4] However, a major tenet of this approach, community participation, is not a distinctly Christian notion; it draws more from democratic and socialist political notions. Proposed modifications to this primary health care approach, an ecological paradigm[5] and a systems approach,[6] are likewise drawn from the academy, not from Christian reflection. Then on the opposite side of the "socialist" primary health care approaches are the individualist free market development notions, not distinctly Christian, used especially by indigenous Pentecostal churches for social ministries of all kinds, including health care.[7]

But are there distinctive Christian approaches? There are certainly approaches drawn from Christian faith. The preferential option for the poor that we considered in Chapter 12 originates in Catholic social teaching. The emphasis on *shalom* ("wholeness") in health is a biblical concept. But again, are these *distinctly* Christian approaches? Or do they even need to be?

At the close of World War II in France, Jacques Ellul

proposed to address the question "What part should [the Christian] play in the life of the world?"[8]—a haunting question in a country compromised and nearly destroyed by the Nazi regime. The question is equally relevant today for Christian global health workers. Ellul begins his response this way:

> …we need to remember that the Christian must not act in exactly the same way as everyone else. He has a part to play in this world which no one else can possibly fulfill. He is not asked to look at the various movements which men have started, choose those which seem "good," and support them…He is charged with a mission of which the natural man can have no idea; yet in reality this mission is decisive for the actions of men.

He then presents three specific biblical functions of Christian engagement in the world:

- To be the salt of the earth: "The fact that Christians *are*, in their lives, the 'salt of the earth,' does far more for the preservation of the world than external action."

- To be the light of the world: "[T]he Christian… reveals to the world the truth about its condition."

- To be sheep in the midst of wolves: "Christians must…offer the daily sacrifice of their lives, which is united with the sacrifice of Jesus Christ."

In all of these functions, Ellul says, we are to be "signs" of the reality of God's action in the world. "Technical work" needs to be done, he says, "but this work is done by everybody, and it has no meaning unless it is guided, accompanied, and sustained by another work that only the Christian can do, and that he often does *not* do." The rest of Ellul's book is an exploration of what this involves.

Ironically—or perhaps understandably—it is a secular study of "humanitarian reason" which most clearly exposes some of what "only the Christian can do." The physician-anthropologist Didier Fassin, in the conclusion to his example-filled study we referred to in Chapter 12, considers the foundations of this humanitarianism.[9] For modern Western societies, he says, engagement with the world is built around how we deal with suffering:

> …while the spectacle of suffering has disappeared completely from the public places where the physical punishment inflicted on criminals was previously exhibited, the representation of suffering through images and narratives has become increasingly commonplace in the public sphere, not only in the media…but also in the political arena, where it furnishes an effective justification for action.

Think of famine, AIDS, and Ebola. He then probes the origins of this focus on suffering:

This fascination with suffering also derives from a Christian genealogy…[T]he valorization of suffering as the basic human experience is closely linked to the passion of Christ redeeming the original sin…The singular feature of Christianity in this respect is that it turns suffering into redemption. However, modernity marks a turning point in this genealogy of redemptive suffering, both in literature and in politics…With the entry of suffering into politics, we might say that salvation emanates not through the passion one endures, but through the compassion one feels.

Humanitarianism has sanitized suffering. This is not the daily sacrifice of our lives, united with the suffering of Christ, of which Ellul wrote. It is not the role of a sheep, but of one who feels sorry for sheep. "In Western societies," writes Fassin, "the paradigm of romantic engagement with the world has thus shifted from the figure of the volunteer risking his or her life alongside liberation movements to the figure of the humanitarian saving lives in spaces set apart from the fighting," spaces he describes a bit later as "protected corridors of aid."

A more disturbing example is a scene from the recent movie *American Sniper*. At a dinner table discussion with his children, one of whom will become the sniper, the father explains to them that there are three types of people in the world: sheep, wolves, and sheepdogs. Sheep, he says, are people who prefer to believe that evil doesn't exist in the world, and if evil presented itself on their doorstep, they wouldn't know how to protect themselves. Wolves are predators who prey on the weak. And sheepdogs are rare: they "are blessed with the gift of aggression" and feel an overwhelming need to protect the flock against wolves. The father was clear: "We aren't raising any sheep in this family...We protect our own." It is the most frightening scene in the movie.

There is no longer any conceptual room for, any understanding of, being sent as sheep in the midst of wolves. Ellul again:

> The world cannot *live* without this living witness of sacrifice. That is why it is essential that Christians should be very careful not to be "wolves" in the spiritual sense— that is, people who try to dominate others. Christians must accept the domination of other people, and offer the daily sacrifice of their lives, which is united with the sacrifice of Jesus Christ.

The world cannot *live* without this kind of sacrifice, and there is something in our humanitarian Western societies that knows this, that remembers this. We knew that Mother Theresa did nothing to prolong the lives of dying people in Calcutta, but we still gave her the Nobel Peace Prize. We knew that three missionaries contracting Ebola did nothing to stop the epidemic, but their story still resonates with something dormant in us. Though it makes no scientific sense, something deep within us *knows* that the world cannot live without this kind of sacrifice. But because it makes no scientific sense, we spend our effort promoting sheepdogs and protected corridors of aid—until a missionary gets Ebola.

Our problem as Christians is that there can be no algorithm for knowing how and when to be preserving salt, revealing light, and especially sheep in the midst of wolves. Ellul admits that we cannot change the world, yet we cannot live with it the way it is. He calls this a "very painful and very uncomfortable situation," yet "we must accept this tension and live in it." And, he says later, "see how God's will of preservation can act in this given situation." The first sacrifice we must make is letting go of the need to control and the assurance of results and of change. It is God's will of preservation, not ours.

Beyond this, there is no formula. For my friend Tom Little, the sacrifice of his life was literal. A Christian optometrist who had worked for over 30 years in Afghanistan, I doubt that he saw living in another culture as a sacrifice. The Tom I knew in college didn't share the upwardly mobile dreams of most students, but he did feel passionate about getting health care to those in rural Afghanistan—and when he and nine other global health workers were killed by the Taliban on the way back from an eye camp in 2010, they died as sheep in the midst of wolves.

For my wife and me, the sacrifice is far more mundane.

Like Tom, we do not find living in Africa for nearly 30 years to be a sacrifice. But as we have moved from working in mission hospitals under mission agencies to working for a public university in a government hospital, we begin to feel more like sheep among wolves. We feel what other staff, and certainly the patients, must feel: in a place where supplies are inadequate, morale is low, and the corruption of politicians sets the example for institutional leadership, services are woefully inadequate. We miss the relative efficiency of mission hospitals, but they have become places to which many patients can no longer go because they cannot afford them. Work for the government is certainly frustrating, but at least we are working with patients who have no other option; at least our view of reality becomes clearer.

We must continue the search for "best practices" for Christian global health workers. We must continue to name our foundations and debate approaches and gather evidence, for we all need to get up in the morning and *do* something. Being salt, light, and sheep among wolves is not a job description; it is who we are, not what we do. But unless we are being what *only* Christians can be, we will have nothing distinctive to offer global health and will play no role in the enlightenment and preservation of the world.

16. Conclusion: Have We Been Invited?

THERE IS A mural in the hospital where I have been working in western Kenya. It's a large mural—about 15 feet by 6 feet—of an African scene: there is a green meadow in the foreground, some hills with trees in the distance, and a blue sky with puffy white clouds. Running through the middle of the picture is a blue river. Beside the river is a single tree, a dead tree with no leaves. A teenage boy has come to cut down the tree with an axe, and has cut out a large wedge, leaving the tree tottering. He hears a lion behind him, and so looks ahead to jump into the river—but finds a crocodile there. His only option is to climb the tottering dead tree, and while climbing we see him dropping his axe. Above his head there is a snake coiled around one branch, flicking his tongue at the boy. On another branch are a beehive and a swarm of those African killer bees.

It's located on a wall just outside the pediatric ward.

This is a global health mural. It tells the story of why global health exists. The only thing missing from the mural are global health workers. That's because global health is still ours—ours in the West, and this is an African mural.

The first global health workers, medical missionaries,

spent a lot of effort trying to rescue that boy from the tree; to *save* him. They had little to work with 200 years ago except their compassion and their prayer. Then science came along—the germ theory, Louis Pasteur, and Robert Koch—and the rescuers began to have some tools to pry him out of that tree. Science gathered momentum.

Waxing and waning throughout the locomotive-like development of this medical science was another approach. One of those scientists, a contemporary of Pasteur and Koch, began to suggest that there were *reasons* that the boy was stuck—social, economic, and political reasons. This was the pathologist Rudolph Virchow. And so was born the *other* approach to global health: fight the lions, kill the crocodiles, exterminate the bees—and in the meantime prop up the tree and feed the boy until we can get him down.

Today our global health projects can be very elaborate: we bring in helicopters with rescue workers who scoop the boy out of the tree, while compassionate commando units tranquilize the lion and crocodile and move them to protected national parks. Then, to prevent the whole scenario from happening again, humbler global health workers develop and distribute solar ovens so the boy won't need to cut firewood any more. We have taken on an enormous task.

But have we been invited to do this task, global health? And if so, by whom? Ollie Fein first illustrated this question to me. I first met Ollie in 1970 in Boston where he was part of a lecture series called Health University—a counter-cultural and counter-political introduction to health care. It was about the American health empire, about community control, about race, about justice. Several years later he would be one of my teachers when I interned at Lincoln Hospital in the Bronx.

But before then, in about 1972, I attended another lecture he was giving somewhere in New York where I was by then a medical student. It was in one of those tiered lecture halls where the podium is way down there in the front. Ollie was talking again about working in underserved areas, and he told us to go and work where the people were organized. Now for me, back then, the word "organize" usually referred to union organizing or political organizing. Ollie's advice bothered me—so in the question time afterward I asked him if he wasn't putting politics ahead of health care with his advice to go only where people were "organized." His answer was not really an answer: he simply said that there are enough communities which are organized.

I hadn't yet realized that he wasn't *just* talking about them being organized; he was also talking about *us* being invited.

I have had several opportunities to ignore Ollie's advice. The first was in 1977. I was near the end of my family medicine residency in Knoxville, Tennessee; I had recently married another doctor, and we were planning to work together. Union County, just north of Knoxville, seemed like a worthy place: 14,000 people, many of them poor, one-third of the homes without indoor plumbing, and no doctor in the county. We visited the public health nurse there, and she told us that the county had a grant for a new community building, so we met the county executive at the building site. It was nearly finished: a multipurpose building housing the local council on aging, the fire department, the employment office, the unemployment office, the library—*and* a doctor's office. "Oh," we said, "a doctor's office? Do you have a doctor planning to come?"

"No."

It seemed like an ideal place for us: a stable, under-served rural community with an empty doctor's office. We talked with the regional public health department and they hired me as the county public health officer; my wife Jan came with the National Health Service Corps. We bought 30 acres of land and a house on the top of Copper Ridge, and eventually had two children. When they came along, we each worked half time…well, two-thirds time. We had a full-service family practice, we shared a job, and we loved the work. We planned to stay forever.

Seven years later we were looking for a new job. Partly we felt a pull to go to Africa—the needs seemed so much greater there. But equally there was a push. Something was wrong, and we're not sure—even now we're not sure—exactly what. We had early on recruited a community board, but it seemed mostly passive, rubber-stamping whatever we suggested. We wanted an active board, so when the terms of the first board were up we hunted around for some more experienced, more active board members. And we got them. They didn't like my flannel shirts; they said I should wear a tie; they told me I should be going to the high school football games. They said we should get to the clinic earlier, even though we first had to make rounds on our inpatients in a Knoxville hospital. Those were just the symptoms of a power struggle we found ourselves embroiled in, one we never intended. We left.

The next chance we had to ignore Ollie's advice was three years later when we were leaving Sudan. We had been working in a Sudanese refugee settlement for Eritreans, doing primary health care; we wanted to work in development, not relief, and return to clinical work—without leaving behind this primary health care. And we found just the place: our agency, a Mennonite organization, had a hospital in Tanzania on Lake Victoria that had recently opened a primary health care department; the two nurses there were doing some interesting community work. *And* the mission compound had a one-room school and a teacher for the missionary children. Everything we wanted. We signed up.

Four years later we broke our contract and left. We

had again shared a job, spending half our time in community work and half in the hospital—while Jan was in the hospital, I was in the community, and vice versa. We gathered all sorts of statistics, did surveys, made some wonderful graphs and maps, and developed a mosquito net program. In the hospital we learned how all the common conditions presented—pneumonia, malaria, diarrhea, obstructed labor, incomplete abortions—and how to treat them. And we learned how to do surgery. But we didn't get along with the doctor in charge, a Tanzanian surgeon, and things got very uncomfortable.

Again, we weren't ready to leave Africa—but we *were* bewildered. Our gallant efforts at primary health care weren't working. The rhetoric was so attractive, but the true community-based programs were hard to find. And we had been so proud of ourselves for working for a Tanzanian doctor, only to find we couldn't get along with him. We had been trying to prop up the tree, chase the lions, exterminate the bees, and also rescue the boy—all under African leadership—and it seemed we had failed.

We didn't know it then, but we had come to the crux of the matter: being invited. We discovered this in retrospect. But during all of our adventures and confusion, we had been gradually discovering that there is much healing wisdom in Africa, and that Africa's acceptance of our Western biomedical "miracles" does not repudiate their own wisdom. I began collecting stories of this healing wisdom, and in the process realized that healing in Africa goes on without us in global health. My metaphor was a wedding, a real wedding of a friend that I had gone to in Tanzania. It was an all-night wedding, and I got sick early in the night and had to go home. The wedding, of course, went on without me. I had the title for my first book.

A few years ago I was telling a professor at Duke University Divinity School about *The Wedding Goes On Without Us*, carried away by my own metaphor, effusing about this wonderful wedding we didn't control, and yet we were invited to it. Professor Emmanuel Katongole, the Ugandan priest who had advised me on some other writings, was standing with us, listening. And then, so kindly, so directly, he looked at me and said, "No, we didn't invite you. You invited yourself." And then the twinkle in his eye: "But we welcomed you." All my attempts at solidarity with Africans up until then got turned upside down. He decided to be in solidarity with me.

We moved to Kenya about 24 years ago and—except for a failed three-year re-entry to the USA—we've lived there ever since. Most of that time we've been in the same area of western Kenya, about half that time in a Quaker mission hospital and the other half with Moi University, trying to develop and teach family medicine. In this job we use the local government hospital for family medicine training, and that is the hospital where we found the mural.

Over the years the patients in our hospital and their visitors have contemplated it, even contributed to it. Occasionally I see mothers, or their children, standing in front of the mural, discussing it. When you look up close now, you see that someone has scratched out the eyes of the crocodile and the lion. I asked the watchman at our home compound why he thought they did this. To him it was simple: the kids were identifying with the boy in the tree and wanted to help him. If the lion and crocodile couldn't see, maybe the boy could jump down and run away.

I too engage with that mural, wondering what it means to the local people who see it, wondering what their lions and crocodiles and bees and snakes are. These are people who have come to this underfunded, sometimes barely functional hospital to be rescued from their own lions and crocodiles, only to find bees and snakes in their place of rescue—a place of relief as precarious as the tree.

A couple years ago my wife saw another child respond to the mural. A small girl, six years old—a patient from the ward with advanced sickle cell disease—was standing in front of the mural, looking up at the boy. She was stretching up to touch the tree and then started jumping, jumping up to try and reach the boy. To touch him, maybe to be with him, maybe to help him. A small girl with advanced sickle cell disease because there was little definitive treatment available for her in our hospital, a girl who knew in those painful bones of hers what the boy was experiencing. The hospital she was depending on was that tottering tree. And all my wife could do is stand there and watch her as she jumped, jumped, reaching....

Epilogue

WE LEFT THE little girl jumping and reaching because global health failed to assist her. On her own she had the energy to enter that tragic mural, to leap toward the boy, to share his plight as he shared hers. That is exactly what she needed then. The best global health could have done is to postpone her jumping and reaching until she was in her twenties, or prevent her from being born.

The tragedy of Onyango, which we began with, has a different lesson. He also had what he needed, but new "*needs*"—material needs created by the same development philosophy that promotes global health—were pulling him away from what he knew, which was that his real strength was in the community of people who would not leave him alone. He was not alone, though for one horrible moment he forgot that. Global health was for him a Trojan horse, smuggling in Western material values.

Both the little girl and Onyango provide silhouettes of truths deeper than global health can penetrate. They had sources of strength and inspiration within their cultures which were—or could have been—vital for their health, sources that global health either ignores or suppresses. It is too busy doing what it set out to do: reducing infant mortality and malnutrition rates, eliminating smallpox and guinea worm and polio, improving vaccination rates, attacking maternal mortality. And when it does well, that success blinds it to everything else. Fortunately smallpox was never a risk for Onyango or the little girl precisely because global health succeeded in eliminating it. But eliminating a disease is not the same as fostering health.

Health means wholeness—the words have the same root—and people are whole only when their physical lives are in harmony with the routine of life in their families and communities. Global health does well in understanding physical lives, because that part is more or less the same throughout the world. But societies and cultures are very different, and global health can only understand these by listening.

Global health that listens is truly global. Global health that does not listen, that reduces health to germs and genes, to biomedical bodies, to statistical progress, is simply the export of the cultural West and the geographic North. It is the most modern, most insidious form of imperialism.

ACKNOWLEDGMENTS

Several of these chapters—or rather pieces or versions of them—were previously published. The early parts of Chapter 1 are from *Bury Me Naked*, a set of stories appended to my first book, *The Wedding Goes On Without Us* (Nairobi, Jacaranda Designs, 2001). Chapter 3 contains Mark Herzog's interview of me, and is used with his permission.

Much of the content of Chapter 5 was first published in the January 21, 2005, issue of the *National Catholic Reporter* as "African Perspective on AIDS Crisis Differs from West." Chapter 6 is an edited version of "HIV/AIDS: Listen to Mbeki," published in Kenya's *Sunday Nation*, November 12, 2000. Chapter 7 is adapted from the prologue to my second book, *As They See It: The Development of the African AIDS Discourse* (London, Adonis and Abbey Publishers, 2005).

Parts of Chapter 13 first appeared in my chapter "ARVs, Morality, and Theology: The Need for Debate," published in *Spirituality for Another Possible World* by Mary N. Getui et al. (Nairobi, Twaweza Communications, 2008). These ideas were also developed in Chapter 8 of my *Death and Life in America: Biblical Healing and Biomedicine* (Scottdale, PA, Herald Press, 2008). Chapter 14 is adapted from "Christian Involvement in Sustainable Development Goals," published in the *Christian Journal for Global Health* (Vol 3, No 1, 2016). A slightly edited version of Chapter 15 appeared as "Should Christian Global Health Be Distinctive?" in the *Christian Journal for Global Health* (Vol 2, No 2, 2015). Chapter 16 was a presentation I gave to a small seminar at Cornell University School of Medicine on April 1, 2015.

NOTES

INTRODUCTION

1. Communication from Dr. Tom Gates.

2. STUCK IN GLOBAL HEALTH

1. See Chapter 6, "Listening to Mbeki."
2. A. Lakoff, "Two Regimes of Global Health" in *Humanity: An International Journal of Human Rights, Humanitarianism, and Development*, Volume 1, Number 1, Fall 2010, pp. 59–79.

4. GLOBAL HEALTH IN HISTORY

1. R. Packard, *A History of Global Health: Interventions Into the Lives of Other Peoples* (Baltimore: Johns Hopkins University Press, 2016).

5. AFRICAN PERSPECTIVES ON AIDS

1. Laurenti Magesa, "Aids and Survival in Africa: A Tentative Reflection," in *Moral and Ethical Issues in African Christianity: A Challenge for African Christianity*, edited by J. N. K. Mugambi and A. Nasimiyu-Wasike (Nairobi: Acton Publishers, 1992, reprinted 2003).

2. L. Magesa, *What is Not Sacred?: African Spirituality* (Nairobi: Acton Publishers, 2014), p. 16.

3. Benezet Bujo, *The Ethical Dimension of Community: The African Model and the Dialogue Between North and South* (Nairobi: Paulines Publications, 1998), Chapter 11.

4. See also Emmanuel Katongole, "Postmodern Illusions and the Challenges of African Theology: The Ecclesial Tactics of Resistance," *Modern Theology* 16:2, April 2000; and "Christian Ethics and AIDS in Africa Today: Exploring the Limits of a Culture of Suspicion and Despair," *Missionalia* 29:2, August 2001, p. 144–160.

6. LISTENING TO MBEKI

1. "Africa Wakes Up to Aids Crisis," *The Guardian Weekly* editorial, July 20–26, 2000, p. 12.

2. Thabo Mbeki, quoted in *Partner: The Newsletter of the Kenyan AIDS NGOs Consortium*, June 2000, p. 2.

3. Oyunga Pala, "A Word from the Editor," *Partner: The Newsletter of the Kenyan AIDS NGOs*, p. 2.

4. Andre Carrel, second letter in "West's Guilt in Aids Despair," *The Guardian Weekly*, July 20–26, 2000, p. 13.

5. http://www.mbeki.org/2016/06/20/remarks-at-the-first-meeting-of-the-presidential-advisory-panel-on-aids-pretoria-20000506/, accessed January 11, 2017.

6. http://www.pbs.org/newshour/bb/africa-jan-june00-mbeki_5-23/, accessed January 11, 2017.

7. http://content.time.com/time/world/article/0,8599,2039809,00.html, accessed January 11, 2017.

8. http://www.virusmyth.com/aids/news/lettermbeki.htm.

9. Jon Cohen, "Companies, Donors Pledge to Close Gap in AIDS Treatment," *Science Magazine*, 289 (5478): 368, July 21, 2000.

10. https://www.standardmedia.co.ke/article/2000229909/donald-trump-shock-for-kenya.

7. WHY IS IT SO DIFFICULT FOR THE WEST TO HEAR AFRICAN VOICES?

1. See multiple examples in R. Downing, *As They See It: The Development of the African AIDS Discourse* (London: Adonis and Abbey, 2005).

2. G. C. Bond et al., *AIDS in Africa and the Caribbean* (Westview Press, 1997), p. xiii.

3. C. Achebe, G. Hyden, C. Magadza, and A. P. Okeyo, *Beyond Hunger in Africa: Conventional Wisdom and an African Vision* (Nairobi: Heinemann Kenya, 1990).

4. Paula Treichler, *How to Have Theory in an Epidemic: Cultural Chronicles of AIDS* (Duke University Press, 1999), pp. 99, 125.

5. E. Kalipeni, S. Craddock, J. Oppong, and J. Ghosh, *HIV and AIDS in Africa: Beyond Epidemiology* (Blackwell Publishing, 2004), pp. 4–5.

6. Solomon Benatar, "Health Care Reform and the Crisis of HIV and AIDS in South Africa," *New England Journal of Medicine* 351:1, pp. 81–92.

7. M. W. Makgoba, "Politics, the Media and Science in HIV/AIDS: the Peril of Pseudoscience," *Vaccine* 20 (2002), pp. 1899–1904.

8. Quoted in the Panos Institute report *Blaming Others: Prejudice, Race, and Worldwide AIDS*, edited by Renee Sabatier (New Society Publishers, 1988), pp. 97–98.

9. V. Y. Mudimbe, *The Invention of Africa: Gnosis, Philosophy, and the Order of Knowledge* (Indiana University Press, 1988), p. 15.

8. LISTENING TO SILENCES

1. Emmanuel Katongole, personal correspondence, January 9, 2005.

2. E. Katongole, "AIDS, Africa and The 'Age of Miraculous Medicine': Naming The Silences, or Recovering an African Theological Voice in the Wake of AIDS and in the Age of Miraculous Medicine" presented at a Catholic Ethics Conference in Padua, Italy, in 2006. A version of the paper, "An Age of Miraculous Medicines," was published as a chapter in B. Bujo and M. Czerny, *AIDS in Africa: Theological Reflections* (Nairobi: Paulines Publications, 2007).

3. E. Fee and N. Krieger, "Understanding AIDS: Historical Interpretations and the Limits of Biomedical Individualism," *American Journal of Public Health* 83:10 (1993), p. 1481.

4. www.anc.org.za/ancdocs/history/mbeki/2000/tm0709.html.

5. Ayi Kwei Armah, *The Healers* (Popenguine, Senegal: Per Ankh, 1978, 2000), p. 262.

6. Ibid., p. 96.

7. Ibid., p. 210.

9. WHAT IS FAMILY MEDICINE IN AFRICA?

1. M. King, *Medical Care in Developing Countries* (Nairobi: Oxford University Press, 1966).

2. Ibid., Preface.

10. MAGESA'S CHALLENGE

1. J. N. K. Mugambi, *Christianity and African Culture* (Nairobi: Acton Publishers, 2002), pp. 152, 154.

2. Ibid., p. 154.

3. Ibid., p. 154.

4. I. R. McWhinney, "Family Medicine in Perspective," *New England Journal of Medicine* 293:4, p. 176–181.

5. Mugambi, p. 161.

6. John Mbiti, *Introduction to African Religion*, second edition
    (Nairobi: East African Educational Publishers, 1991), p. 175.

7. Ibid., p. 174.

8. Benezet Bujo, *The Ethical Dimension of Community: The African
    Model and the Dialogue Between North and South* (Paulines
    Publications Africa, 1998), pp. 181–195.

9. Laurenti Magesa, "Aids and Survival in Africa: A Tentative
    Reflection," in *Moral and Ethical Issues in African Christianity: A
    Challenge for African Christianity*, edited by J. N. K. Mugambi
    and A. Nasimiyu-Wasike (Nairobi: Acton Publishers, 1992,
    reprinted 2003), pp. 197–216.

11. FAMILY MEDICINE RESEARCH

1. R. Mash, R. Downing, S. Moosa, and J. De Maeseneer,
    "Exploring the Key Principles of Family Medicine in Sub-Saharan
    Africa: International Delphi Consensus Process," *SA Fam Pract*
    2008; 50(3), pp. 60–65.

2. S. Reid, R. Mash, R. Downing, and S. Moosa, "Perspectives on
    Key Principles of Generalist Medical Practice in Public Service in
    Sub-Saharan Africa: A Qualitative Study," *BMC Family Practice*
    2011, 12:67.

3. S. Moosa, R. Downing, R. Mash, S. Reid, S. Pentz, and A.
    Essuman, "Understanding of Family Medicine in Africa: A
    Qualitative Study of Leaders' Views," *British Journal of General
    Practice* 2013; 63, pp. 139–140.

12. THE CHRISTIAN ROOTS OF GLOBAL HEALTH

1. D. Fassin, *Humanitarian Reason: A Moral History of the Present*
    (Berkeley: University of California Press, 2012), p. 248.

2. Ibid., p. 249.

3. M. Griffin and J. Weiss Block, eds., *In the Company of the Poor: Conversations with Dr. Paul Farmer and Fr. Gustavo Gutierrez* (Maryknoll, NY: Orbis Books, 2013), p. 7ff.

4. Ibid.

5. Ibid., p. 16.

6. Ibid., Chapter 5.

7. Ibid., p. 150.

8. J. Ellul, *Presence in the Modern World*, translated by Lisa Richmond (Eugene, Oregon: Cascade Books, Wipf and Stock, 2016), pp. 8–9, 63–64 (this is a new translation of *The Presence of the Kingdom*).

13. JUSTICE AND LISTENING

1. P. Farmer et al., *Reimagining Global Health: An Introduction* (Berkeley: University of California Press, 2013), p. 111. Randall Packard also links the origins of global health to AIDS; he has a chapter in *A History of Global Health* entitled "AIDS and the Birth of Global Health."

2. Ivan Illich, "Missionary Poverty," in *The Church, Change, and Community Development* (out of print); chapter available at http://englewoodreview.org/ excerpt-ivan-illich-on-missional-poverty-vol-2-14/.

3. Ivan Illich, "The Eloquence of Silence," in *Celebration of Awareness* (Garden City, New York: Doubleday & Co., 1970), p. 50.

14. DEVELOPMENT IN BABYLON

1. http://www.undp.org/content/undp/en/home/mdgoverview.
html.

2. Revelation 21:1–4; 18:7.

3. Leviticus 19:10; Psalm 9:12, 41:1, 68:10, 72:2ff, 82:3–4, 112:9,
113:7, 132:15; Proverbs 14:21,31, 19:17, 22:9, 28:29, 31:9;
Isaiah 1:17; Luke 7:22; James 5:4.

4. http://journal.cjgh.org/index.php/cjgh/issue/view/13.

5. "The 2030 Agenda comprises 17 new Sustainable Development
Goals (SDGs), or Global Goals, which will guide policy and
funding for the next 15 years, beginning with a historic pledge
to end poverty. Everywhere. Permanently." http://www.undp.
org/content/undp/en/home/mdgoverview.html.

6. This brief discussion is drawn from the arguments fully
developed in *The Development Dictionary*, edited by Wolfgang
Sachs. The new edition is available for free download at https://
www.google.com/search?client=ubuntu&channel=fs&q=Sachs+
The+Development+Dictionary&ie=utf-8&oe=utf-8.

7. J. Ellul, *The Technological Society* (Alfred Knopf, 1964).

8. "The condition at the end of time which today takes its form
in our thoughts, feelings, and perceptions—can only be
grasped by those who unequivocally believe in the reality of
the Gospel." B. Duden, quoting Illich in "Ivan Illich—Beyond
Medical Nemesis (1976): The Search for Modernity's
Disembodiment of 'I' and 'You,'" available at www.pudel.
uni-bremen.de/pdf/lv_tra_b.pdf. "I could not have analyzed
medicine without bringing into this analysis my passionate
attempt to understand a little bit of the Gospels…" Illich, in
David Cayley, ed., *The Rivers North of the Future* (Anansi Press,
2005), p. 121.

9. Ivan Illich, *In the Mirror of the Past* (London: Marion Boyars
Publishers, 1992), pp. 21–2.

10. Ivan Illich, *Celebration of Awareness* (Doubleday and Co., 1970), pp. 165, 159, 23.

11. http://news.yahoo.com/richest-62-people-control-same-wealth-poorest-half-165238838--abc-news-topstories.html.

12. http://finance.yahoo.com/news/stark-inequality-oxfam-says-8-000245568.html.

13. J. Ellul, *The Presence of the Kingdom* (Seabury Press, 1967), Chapter III "The Ends and the Means."

15. GLOBAL HEALTH: IS SUFFERING NECESSARY?

1. M. A. Strand and A. M. Cole, "Framing the Role of the Faith Community in Global Health," *Christian Journal for Global Health* 1(2):7–15. http://journal.cjgh.org/cjgh/index.php/cjgh/article/view/19/109.

2. R. Downing, "The Gospel of Health," *Christian Journal for Global Health* 2(1):43–48. http://journal.cjgh.org/cjgh/index.php/cjgh/article/download/25/190.

3. S. Litsios, "The Christian Medical Commission and the Development of the World Health Organization's Primary Health Care Approach," *Am J Public Health* 2004 Nov;94(11):1884–1893. http://ajph.aphapublications.org/doi/abs/10.2105/AJPH.94.11.1884.

4. J. M. De Angulo and L. S. Losada, "Health Paradigm Shifts in the 20th Century," *Christian Journal for Global Health* 2(1):49–58. http://journal.cjgh.org/cjgh/index.php/cjgh/article/download/37/191.

5. Ibid.

6. R. C. Swanson and B. J. Thacker, "Systems Thinking in Short-term Health Missions: A Conceptual Introduction and Consideration of Implications for Practice," *Christian Journal for Global Health* 2(1):7–22. http://journal.cjgh.org/cjgh/index.php/cjgh/article/download/50/192.

7. B. L. Myers, "Progressive Pentecostalism, Development, and Christian Development NGOs: A Challenge and an Opportunity," *Int BMs Res.* 1915 Jul;39(3):115–120.

8. J. Ellul, *The Presence of the Kingdom*, first edition (New York: Seabury Press, 1967) [first edition in French 1948]. All quotes from the first chapter, "The Christian in the World."

9. D. Fassin, *Humanitarian Reason: A Moral History of the Present* (Berkeley: University of California Press, 2012). All quotes from the Conclusion.